Drinking Problems
at the Fountain of Youth

ALSO BY BETH TEITELL

From Here to Maternity:
The Education of a Rookie Mom

Drinking Problems at the Fountain of Youth

Beth Teitell

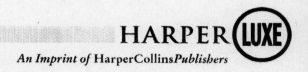

HARPER LUXE

An Imprint of HarperCollinsPublishers

HarperCollins books may be purchased for educational, business, or sales promotional use. For information please write: Special Markets Department, HarperCollins Publishers, 10 East 53rd Street, New York, NY 10022.

FIRST HARPERLUXE EDITION

HarperLuxe™ is a trademark of HarperCollins Publishers

Library of Congress Cataloging-in-Publication Data is available upon request.

ISBN: 978-0-06-166818-0

08 09 10 11 12 ID/RRD 10 9 8 7 6 5 4 3 2 1

You're never too old
to become younger.

—MAE WEST

Contents

Introduction: Defining, Defying, Denying:
The New Age   1

1. Einstein's Theory of Relativity as Applied
   to Crow's-Feet   8

2. Older Women, Younger Shirts   28

3. Pore, Pore, Pitiful Me   46

4. Post-Traumatic Tress Disorder   67

5. Age Is the New Fat   85

6. The Absolute(ish) Truth   102

7. How to Look "Natural" in Three
   Hours or Less   119

8. Facial Fitness: No Pain, No Vain   135

9. Face Value   154

10. Did She or Didn't She?   170

11. The Middle-aged Debutante 188
12. Don't Call Me Ma'am! 207
13. What Lies Beneath 223
14. You've Come a Long Way, Laddie 238
   Conclusion: Carpe Dermis 247

   Acknowledgments 261

Introduction

Defining, Defying, Denying: The New Age

*Time is a great healer but
a lousy beautician.*
—ANONYMOUS

Ladies, brace yourselves. There's a war afoot, a War on Aging, and hostilities are escalating. Our life spans are lengthening, but we're stressing about looking old ever younger. Yes, forty is the new thirty, but little good it does us. As you may have heard, it's also the case that thirty is the new forty. It's never too early for a preventive procedure—or five. These days, trying to appear young is a full-time job, with no vacation allowed. There are muscles to lean and lengthen, antiaging hair masques to apply, youthful yet age-appropriate clothing to buy, non-oldies music to listen to. If I could reclaim the years I've spent perking my rear, I'd actually be the age I'm trying to feign.

Then what, I'm not sure, but I do know this: to ignore your cosmetic-improvement options—to give in to vertical lip lines and "mom jeans" and reading glasses—is to admit defeat and fall behind, to be mistaken for a woman your own age. The shame.

Like millions of other women under crushing pressure to stem time's ravages, I approach each day as if I were at spa boot camp. If I'm doing things right, I'll look younger today than I did yesterday, and even more youthful tomorrow. By the end of the week, I'll be carded while trying to buy Shiraz. Who's barking out the orders? The Cosmeceutical-Industrial Complex? The Gap? *Us Weekly?* Ourselves? Our husbands? Friends? Enemies? Bosses? Big Botox? All of the above? Whoever it is, the message is as sharp as your dead skin cells are dull: Age at your own risk.

We may look better, in a lineless, poreless, expressionless way, but this youth-and/or-bust imperative exacts a psychological toll. It makes normal women—academics, housewives, nonprofit executives, for goodness' sake—feel they need to be as camera-ready as actresses and newscasters, and, worse, as insecure and vulnerable to advertising as they were back in high school. Twenty years after Christie Brinkley sucked me in during her first stint as a Cover Girl, convincing me that with the right foundation I could look just like her—a mask, wig, and body double would have been more like it—she's wooing me again with an Advanced Radiance Age Defying line. Christie, please, take pity. Just when I'd finally gotten my body image and self-esteem issues under control, here you are again, turning me into an age-orexic.

Years ago, covering the Miss America Pageant for the *Boston Herald,* I discovered the frightening concept of "aging out." That's what happens to "girls" who get too old to compete for the crown. At twenty-four, they age out of the system. At least back then I thought only beauty queens were at risk; now I realize that we're all Miss Altoona. It's just that if you're not parading around in a bathing suit and a sash, the dividing line isn't quite so absolute. The cute sales associate at J. Crew won't confiscate the skimpy sundress you're trying to purchase, but make no mistake: The "sell by" date on your "miss" years is etched on your forehead all the same.

I learn my lesson every single "ma'am" day. As in: "Did you find everything you were looking for today, ma'am?"

Yes, except how to "defy" my age, as the multi-billion-dollar cosmeceuticals industry commands.

There's Christie's Cover Girl line, of course, Olay's Age Defying Revitalizing Eye Gel, Keri's Age Defy and Protect Moisture Therapy, A-Defiance from Serious Skin Care, Ponds age defEYEs, and so many others that it almost defies belief. Otherwise mentally sound women are turning into junkies, so desperate to defy Mother Nature—the bee-yotch—that we're willing to risk our health and even our lives for the high of shaving a few years off our appearance. As one homemaker confided: "I'm always thinking about when I can get my Botox fix."

I'm always considering miracle procedures, too, okay, I obsess about them—but I won't go the nip-and-prick route. At least I hope not. "Why the hell not?" a friend asked, as baffled as if I'd opted for a Novocain-free root canal. "Is it not wanting, on principle, to be part of the Plastic Generation?" Ethically, I have nothing against mid-brow lifts and tummy tucks—unless a friend is getting them, which makes *me* look older by comparison, and then I'm aghast at her shallowness. It's more that I'm not willing to risk the complications of "elective" surgery. The War on Aging is not without casualties. Every day—or at least every new issue of a women's magazine or the Thursday and Sunday *New York Times* Styles sections—brings grim news from the front. Friendly fire it ain't. Women are suffering Thermage burns, liposuction indentations, bunching from thread face-lifts, the dreaded "trout pout." I recently learned that a botched nose job can destroy your sense of smell. And with procedures running in the thousands of dollars, and many only temporary in nature, expense is also a major deterrent. Lending companies *do* offer financing options, but at rates that hit almost 28 percent if you're a bad risk (for repayment, not for looking better). And continuing to make loan payments long after your eyelids have resagged is like paying off your fantasy wedding years after you've divorced. Totally pathetic.

But of course it's not just your face on which you must lavish funds. The older you get, the more important you consider the supporting players: hair, handbags, shoes, anything capable of diverting attention from the problem area. You may want to carry a small dog. Dress and grooming that are fine for twenty-year-olds—minimal amounts of sheer clothing, unpainted nails, unkempt hair—make the forty-year-old look like she's off her meds. The investment of time, money, and product it takes simply to appear well rested (a look no longer achievable through actual sleep) is mind-boggling. Alas, if only there were a federal ma'am-icare program to cover the cost of this "disease"—fear of looking our age—that we've caught from society. And while we're at it, in addition to maternity leave, which not every woman takes anyway, employers should grant "facial leave." I could sure use the time. My morning microdermabrasing-cleansing-clarifying-restoring-reversing-rejuvenating-regenerating-refining-replenishing-renewing-brightening-tightening-toning-lifting-lightening-hydrating-protecting-defending-defining-defying-correcting-concealing-smoothing-plumping-minimizing routine takes so long that when I'm done it's almost night, and time to begin the ritual again. Then I lie awake at 3 A.M., worrying that I'm exfoliating the very skin I'm paying a fortune to moisturize.

When I couldn't sleep the other night, I grabbed the Bliss catalog from my nightstand, where it sits atop my other favorite literature: *New Beauty* magazine's "age defying" issue and the latest issue of SkinStore.com's catalog. Big mistake. Bliss was telling tales of serums that erase dark under-eye circles, exfoliation systems that can bring back taut mid-twenties skin, creams that erase vertical lip lines. I couldn't stop turning the pages. It was like reading porn—only more exciting. By the time I got to the part about Lift Fusion, a topical face-lift that uses a "breakthrough M-Tox technology to make all forms of furrows visibly vamoose," not only was I flushed, but I knew I had to visit this little hottie in person. The next day I hit Sephora on my way to work and slathered on as much Lift Fusion ($140 per 1.75 ounces) as possible before a saleswoman headed over with the dreaded "Can I help you?" "I'm all set," I said, my booty practically dripping from my face. I couldn't wait to see the new me in the mirror. Alas, she looked exactly like the old me, but who was *I* to judge? Or, as Chico Marx once asked: "Who are you going to believe? Me, or your own eyes?"

With a nod to Chico, this book chronicles my quest to answer *the* question of our skin-deep times: Short of minimally or maximally invasive procedures, is there anything out there that actually helps? Are yoga facials the secret? Do $25-per-bag "skin-gestible" gummi bears truly tighten pores? (Binge on those babies and you'll look like a chubby teenager.) Is it all about concealer? Should I change my name to something less middle-agey-sounding? Caitlin, maybe?

"I'm a woman on the verge," I told my husband, Ken, the other day, when the madness started to get the best of me. "On the verge of what?" he asked.

Looking younger or older. I'm not sure which.

1.

Einstein's Theory of Relativity as Applied to Crow's-Feet

Every time a friend succeeds, I die a little.
—GORE VIDAL

Friends don't let friends undergo minimally or maximally invasive procedures. Why? Because every wrinkle your friend freezes, every jowl she tightens, every crease she plumps, only throws your own imperfections into greater relief. It's like Einstein said: Space and time are relative, rather than absolute, concepts. In appearance terms, his theory of relativity means that the younger those around you look, the older you do. Okay, Einstein himself never said that exactly, but you've seen pictures of the man; I'm sure he'd agree.

The problem is that life's one big bell curve and some of us are ruining it for the rest of us. (You know who you are.) It doesn't take an Einstein to see what's happening to those too risk-averse, financially challenged, delusional, or complacent to go under the knife. We're being shoved into an emerging and highly undesirable demographic: the "cosmetic underclass."

This sad new group of victims was identified in a 1996 article in the London *Times*. A mere four years after the Environmental Protection Agency concluded that exposure to secondhand smoke presented a serious public health threat, the dangers of passive cosmetic surgery were also recognized. "Disfigurement is the last bastion of discrimination," Gus McGrouther, Britain's first professor of plastic surgery, told the paper. The article went on to question "where imperfection stops and deformity begins. With our cheque books, probably."

And how prophetic that story was: as matters now stand, you needn't have a procedure to put yourself at risk. Mere proximity to someone artificially enhanced is harmful—to your ego. We've got to do something to slow the trend. Statistics from the American Society for Aesthetic Plastic Surgery show that 2.1 million cosmetic surgical and 9.6 million cosmetic nonsurgical procedures were performed in the United States in 2007. Once you remove the kids and the guys from the population count, that's something like one procedure for every ten women. Or worse. In beauty danger zones like Miami, the Upper East Side, and Beverly Hills, it's probably closer to ten procedures for every one woman. And those 11.7 million procedures represent a whopping 457 percent increase since the group began collecting such statistics in 1997. The Centers for Disease Control hasn't used the word, but it's clear we've got an epidemic on our hands.

No one's safe. Not even the rich. I know women who studied hard to get into good colleges, worked their connections to land enviable jobs, married well, produced children who could pose for Ralph Lauren ads, vacation on the right islands with the right beach towels and the right heiresses—they have fractional ownerships in Cessnas, for heaven's sake—and yet if they have furrows and hints of upper-lip lines and puppet mouth when those around them are smoother than freshly ironed Pratesi linens, what's it all worth? In a word, nothing.

Self-help experts always advise against comparing yourself to others, and it's wise counsel. I pass it on to my kids all the time. But what happens when you accept your position in the appearance pecking order— you're not the most youthful fifty-year-old around, say, but not the most aged, either—only to find that you *are* the old crone? That while you've been foolishly priding yourself on "aging naturally"—there's a retronym for you—others have been slipping off to the dermatologist's office. By staying still, you can actually be moving backward.

Unfortunately, I'm speaking from personal experience. The following tale doesn't make me look good, but then again, that's the whole problem, isn't it? A woman I've known since we were both dewy twenty-somethings (and didn't appreciate how good we had it) recently informed me of her decision to Botox her brow furrows. I love her like a sister, so *of course* I want her to look her best, but from my perspective, her unilateral move was an obvious violation of our (admittedly) unspoken treaty to age at the same rate. She pulled the beauty equivalent of doping, and in this scenario I'm the athlete who's playing by the rules and being penalized. It gives me even more sympathy for Tour de France cyclists and baseball players competing without pharmaceutical help. We should start testing civilians for appearance-enhancing drugs.

I'm not trying to claim I was thrilled with the way I was aging before my pal pulled her fast one, but prior to her little trip to the doctor, procedures, like weekend jaunts to Paris, and Hermès Birkin bags, hadn't penetrated my inner circle. Surgery and injectables were all available, but I was an onlooker, not a potential participant. I didn't consider myself the *kind of person* who has work done. Actually, let me clarify that: I'm not the *kind of person* who thinks there's a *kind of person* who has work done. That's too judgmental, which I'm not. Just sort of jealous—and sort of disappointed that options have become available. Nothing's more stressful than missing an opportunity you wish didn't exist.

I'll never forget that cold, cold day in August when my friend called and, twenty minutes into our chat, just happened to mention that she'd Done It.

There was no "Sit down, I have some difficult news," no "I hope this doesn't come between us." She lives just a few blocks from me, but she didn't even pay me the courtesy of telling me face-to-face, although, to be fair, that might have been even more upsetting, as my brow wrinkled in horror and hers stayed enviably smooth.

"What?" I said, sick to my stomach. "Why didn't you tell me?"

"I just did."

Technically, she was right. I guess what I meant was: "Why didn't you consult me beforehand so I could scare you out of it, under the guise of concern over potential side effects?"

I ran to my bathroom mirror. Wrinkles that had been merely disappointing were now unbearable. Over the course of a few seconds, I'd aged twenty years. What had I been thinking, letting myself go like this? "You must look great!" I said tightly, not even adding our usual disclaimer, "Not that you needed it."

Why am I so threatened? It's not that I don't want my friend (who'd crossed from the Furrowed to the Smoothie camp overnight) to be happy. It's just that, well . . . let's just say a study by two Arizona State University psychologists sums up my feelings: women who are surrounded by other attractive women, the researchers found, report being less secure of their appearance than those wise enough to hang with ugly ducklings. "If there are a large number of desirable members of one's own sex available, one may regard one's own market value as lower," the researchers reported in the *Personality and Social Psychology Bulletin*.

And you know what stinks? The less attractive women are *right* to feel that way. Of the many studies confirming the existence of the so-called contrast effect, my favorite is the one in which male dormitory residents are shown an episode of *Charlie's Angels* and then asked to rate a photo of an average female (described to them by researchers as a potential blind date for another dorm resident). Well, well, well. Guess what? These subjects rated the "target female" as "significantly less attractive" than did a comparable control group not forced to watch the show, the study reported.

Actually, suffering in comparison to actresses I can deal with. My defense mechanisms are so well developed that I've convinced myself they're probably shallow and unhappy. What bothers me is being a lot less attractive than my own friends. But here's where anti-aging "advances" make things hard: You bond with an equally lined and wrinkled woman, and then she pulls a bait and switch and becomes a Fountainista, throwing the friendship math out of whack. Because despite the *Charlie's Angels* findings, your true competitors aren't the boldfaced names in *People* and *Us Weekly,* but rather the people who subscribe to those magazines. David Buss, an evolutionary psychologist from the University of Texas who studies envy, explained that we generally measure ourselves against a "relevant reference group." This behavior dates to a time long ago (before anyone had heard of Farrah Fawcett), when small-group living meant our competitors were in our immediate environment.

It's this phenomenon, Buss told me, that makes us envy a house slightly nicer than the one we can afford, but not one way out of our league, like Donald Trump's. The professor didn't make a link between real estate envy and appearance envy, but one of my friends—super funny, *super* covetous—sure did. "I get jealous of cosmetic surgery the way I get jealous of people I know who were smart enough to invest in a condo in the South End years ago," she said, referring to the gentrified Boston neighborhood. "In both cases, they're already so far ahead of me, and will be even better off ten years from now—when I'll be broke and my boobs will be doubling as fanny packs."

I'm not proud of my envy, but at least I'm not at the point where I'm begrudging my own mother cosmetic enhancement (okay, she hasn't had any). But cosmetic procedures have so infected society that they are starting to strain even the closest of blood relations. Consider this letter to an advice columnist: "My 53-year-old mom discovered plastic surgery a few years ago, and now she looks younger than I do (I'm 27)," "D.C. from Texas" wrote to *USA Weekend* in May 2006. "Everyone—including my husband—has commented on how great she looks and how she now looks more like my sister than my mother. I know it shouldn't, but the constant comparison, even from her, is driving me crazy! Why is this getting to me? Also, how should I handle the next annoying comment about how old and tired I look next to her?"

The answer? "First, you should stop thinking of compliments to her as digs at you. You need to end the competition and comparison, and find joy in her happiness. . . . You shouldn't feel bad about your feelings, however. Just as it's natural for your mother to seek beauty validation, it's human nature for you to feel jealous—even of your mother."

D.C.'s letter prompted me to survey daughters, and such feelings turn out to be more common than you'd think. "My mother saddled me with this schnozz and then goes and gets hers bobbed off," one woman wrote. Another admitted jealously eyeing her mom's newly smooth décolletage. We can only hope that one day doctors will come up with a way for cosmetic surgery enhancements to be passed along in the genes. If mom gets a boob job, her daughters will be born big-busted. It would be the modern version of Lamarckian evolution, the nineteenth-century idea that a living being can pass on characteristics acquired during its lifetime to its offspring.

I figured that few daughters would have more to say on the subject than Melissa Rivers, and as luck would have it, she and Joan were performing at the AARP convention in Boston in a ballroom that held four thousand people. Okay, let me stop right here and answer the question that every single person asks when she hears I saw Joan. How did she look? Just like she does on TV: a platinum head atop a windblown face atop a stick body. She and Melissa had the crowd laughing for an hour, and then took questions. "Melissa," I yelled out, "are you worried that your mother's going to start looking younger than you do?" "No," she replied. "I'm just concerned that I have to keep reintroducing her to my son." As the crowd cracked up, Joan called out in a raspy yell: "They call me 'Nana New Face.'"

It's been a while since I learned of my friend's cosmetic treachery, and although it eats at me, I've yet to go in for a "defensive" procedure myself, although I fear it may be only a matter of time. When I told Valerie Monroe, the beauty director of *O* magazine, about my mixed feelings—I don't want to have work but I don't want others to gain an advantage—she said she often hears similar ambivalence from her readers. They don't want to "muck" with what they have, but they're concerned that "a lot of people are getting stuff done, and if you don't are you losing out? Are you not doing the best thing for yourself? What I don't see enough of," she added, "and what I wish I saw more of, were emails from women who are accepting the changes [of age]. But it's very difficult."

Wouldn't it be great if we could all sign a nonproliferation, noninjectable pact? I won't do anything if you don't. As matters now stand, we're on a course of mutually assured exhaustion, leading where, I'm not sure. But I'm not getting my hopes up for any de-escalation. As one cosmetic surgery consultant— yes, that's a real job—told me, "If you belong to a social set and all of a sudden you're the 'oldest' woman at the table, you'd better catch up, even if you're the type who wouldn't be inclined." That was Wendy Lewis talking. She's the famed "Knife Coach" of Manhattan and London. Clients pay her $400 per hour to advise them on what work they need and who might do it. That's "need" as in "I need that Marc Jacobs bag," not "I need to have a tooth pulled." Although as society becomes ever more appearance-focused, with all the good jobs and the best mates going to the nipped and tucked, opting out may become a liability. One may actually *need* a lift.

I don't like to say that, but it may be true. While many studies have shown that better-looking people get better jobs, get paid more, etc., a first-of-its-kind study found that the same benefits accrue to those who've had plastic surgery. Writing in the October 2004 issue of the medical journal *Aesthetic Plastic Surgery*, the researchers claim their work "scientifically validates that plastic surgery can enhance the first impression that one makes." Randomly selected unknowing observers separately evaluated before and after photographs of patients who had undergone facial cosmetic surgery, they explained, and the findings indicated that after facial cosmetic surgery patients were graded as 31 percent more attractive, 27 percent greater in social skills, 22 percent higher in dating success, 19 percent better in athletic skills, 15 percent higher in relationship skills, and 13 percent higher in financial success.

But the real significance of the study, according to the principle investigator, was that the positive effects of plastic surgery did not derive solely from the enhanced self-confidence of the patients. "I am often told by my patients that following their cosmetic surgery procedure they have achieved a new job, an improved romantic relationship or greater personal success," Dr. Steven H. Dayan, a clinical assistant professor at the University of Illinois School of Medicine, wrote. "I had always felt that it was secondary to a greater self confidence which had projected through, but I now have to consider that maybe there is more to it."

As for me, I was relieved that I was talking to Lewis, the cosmetic surgery consultant, over the phone, not in her Upper East Side office. How could I have conducted an interview knowing that she'd note every expression line or double chin I set off with a smile or eyebrow raise? But Lewis wasn't about to let me off so easy. "Send me a picture of yourself," she said. She'd do an analysis—free! I begged off and felt pretty happy about dodging a bullet, only to come face-to-face with her a few weeks later, at the Health & Beauty America convention in New York (a meeting whose attendees were so focused on appearance that the lines in the ladies' room were not for the toilets, but for the mirrors).

Lewis was moderating a panel on trends in cosmetic surgery—a topical Botox-like product that *works* is coming, but it's years and years off—and afterward I went up and introduced myself, making sure we were in a dark corner and my hair was covering as much of my face as possible without making me look deranged. "Okay," I said, confronting the inevitable, "tell me what I need to have done." "We need better light," she said, brushing my hair from my face. I braced myself for her diagnosis: Botox for crow's-feet would help, and I *must* do something for my lips. She was trying to be nice, I could tell, but as a healer she had an obligation to alert me to what was threatening to become a bad situation. "They're very very dry," she said. "I can see lines. What do you use to moisturize them?"

"My tongue."

Yes, I scoured Manhattan for the $50 lip exfoliation system Lewis recommended. When I got back to Boston I thought that maybe it was time to take my flirtation with Botox to the next level—to make our relationship physical. If only it weren't for Ken, my beloved, my soul mate, the person standing between me and real happiness! For the past few years, I'd been battling not just my own reluctance to have anything done, but his. He's a doctor, but a pediatrician, darn it, not a plastic surgeon, and as a health care professional he's all too aware of what can go wrong, even though I'd explained to him many times that a procedure done in a mall, next to a Cinnabon kiosk, isn't truly "medical."

I certainly wouldn't say Botox has become a problem in our relationship, but disagreement over cosmetic procedures can cause stress, according to the marriage and family therapists I spoke with. Dr. Gail Saltz, the psychiatrist, author, and TV commentator, told me she sees pressure coming from both sides. Sometimes husbands want wives to get breast implants, and the wives pretty easily "succumb." "Would that this were not the case," Saltz said, "but most women don't have so much confidence in their own bodies." While men wanting bustier wives is the cliché, the more common scenario, Saltz told me, is when the woman wants to do her lips, or get a tummy tuck or have lipo, and "the husband's like, 'Who's that for? Not for me. I like you the way you are.' A lot of women get cosmetic surgery not for men or even themselves but other women. Women are very competitive." The men, she added, are often concerned about cost, safety, and added responsibilities during the wife's recovery time. The threat of having to do laundry and grocery shop, it seems, is up there with fear over anesthesia complications.

In fact, an "American Pulse" poll conducted by BIGresearch, the consumer marketing firm, found that only 2.8 percent of men would encourage a spouse or significant other to have surgery or a procedure. That number's not high, but, I might note, it is larger than the number for females. Only 1.9 percent of women said they'd do the same.

Using all my feminine wiles, I cooked Ken a nice dinner and applied lipstick (as if I were a housewife from the 1950s, but those poor dears, having to make do without topical lip plumpers). But rather than dim the lights, I brightened them, the better to illustrate my point. "I'm getting Botox," I said, caressing his face and bracing for an argument.

I could tell he was eager to present me with documented cases of bad outcomes, but he knew me better than to resort to facts. He went with the I-love-you-just-the-way-you-are defense: "But you look great already," he offered. *Awwww.* That sounds so sweet, doesn't it? But deep down—where more wrinkles were already forming as the fat cells in my subcutaneous layer shrink—I saw his flattery for what it was: less loving endorsement than the caution of a regular reader of the Centers for Disease Control's *Morbidity and Mortality Weekly Report.*

"I don't even know where you'd need it," he tried. You'll of course recognize this as a variation on the "No, it doesn't make you look fat" line of a man fearful of wandering into dangerous waters. Just as only an idiot points to her saddlebags and says "Here's the cellulite I'm always complaining about" to a guy she's dating, a wife *does not* point out which areas need work (on the very off chance he truly hadn't noticed).

"You should be happy he loves you as is," a colleague who Botoxes said. *Her* husband, she complained, is too supportive. "He was so enthusiastic that even if I didn't want to keep doing it I'd have to."

But of course there's no way she's giving up her quarterly facial refreshers. "I couldn't go back to doing nothing," she admitted. "The Botoxed me has become the real me, to the point where the person with wrinkles—I don't know who she is."

I do. She's *me,* that's who. Not to sound bitter, but my friend's satisfaction with her work is a perfect illustration of the observation made in the Spring 2004 issue of the *New Atlantis* magazine. "Cosmetic surgery might make individual people happier, but in the aggregate it makes life worse for everyone."

That struck such a note that I called the author, Christine Rosen, a fellow at the Washington-based Ethics and Public Policy Center. She likened getting plastic surgery to driving an SUV. Good for the owner, but bad not only for the environment but also for other drivers who are forced to get their own large, gas-guzzling vehicles out of self-defense. With ever more people having work done, Rosen worries about the potential for "beauty pollution." She was only partially joking when she suggested people start thinking about their "Juvederm footprints." What an idea! If only users were required to submit to the beauty equivalent of carbon offsets. Let's see, you're having your nasolabial folds taken care of, so no getting your hair professionally blow-dried for three months.

But that's a pipe dream. Here's the reality: the more people who have plastic surgery, the more people who need to have plastic surgery. Abigail Brooks, a visiting assistant professor in sociology at Boston College, whose 2007 dissertation was on "Growing Older in a 'Surgical Age': An Analysis of Women's Lived

Experiences and Interpretations of Aging in an Era of Cosmetic Surgery," says her data "reveals that the more women are exposed to these antiaging surgeries and technologies, the worse they feel about their own aging faces and bodies, hence the increased likelihood that they themselves will have and use these anti-aging surgeries and technologies."

Brooks worries that we are "shrinking our potential to think of beauty in diverse ways" and "narrowing the beauty cannon." As she puts it: "We're losing our ability to define beauty outside the physical range."

Similarly, Kathryn Pauly Morgan, the feminist philosopher, has identified a "technological beauty imperative." "Now technology is making obligatory the appearance of youth and the reality of 'beauty' for every woman who can afford it," she writes in *Women and the Knife: Cosmetic Surgery and the Colonization of Women's Bodies.* "Natural destiny is being supplanted by technologically grounded coercion, and the coercion is camouflaged by the language of choice, fulfillment, and liberation."

And fight it at your own risk. As a social historian, Lynne Luciano Loeb, an associate professor of history at California State University, Dominguez Hills, told me: "If you don't continue to try to look young, it sort of implies you've given up. Keeping up used to be wearing new styles; now it means how much effort are you putting into making yourself look younger."

As a society, we've gone from liberation—older people don't have to feel or act old—to repression—you *can't* be old. Because Americans marry later and more often than in the past, change jobs more frequently, post pictures of ourselves on the web and appear in YouTube videos, we're essentially on the market our whole adult lives. "People are so much more in the public eye than they've ever been," Loeb said. And thanks to digital cameras with their horrible display screens, we also see *ourselves* more, too—and in real time.

As Loeb spoke, I thought about how much better my newbie Smoothie friend will look than I do, and I was overcome with the unfairness of it all. "I'm doing it!" I told Ken a few weeks later. "No you're not," he said. "You're not the boss of me!" I yelled.

"Why tell him?" a friend asked. I'd thought of that, but the implications frightened me. Sneaking in a Bloomingdale's bag is one thing, but surreptitious Botox? If he didn't detect it, what would that say about how much attention he pays? And yet, how could I justifiably accuse him of *not* noticing? "I secretly did something you don't agree with and you didn't even spot it!" It's a hard case to make, even by my own double standards. And besides, what if there were side effects (besides a loss of trust)? "Uh, honey, I know I didn't mention I was going in for a procedure, but well, I did, and now I'm in the emergency room." It could get awkward.

Actually, even if he changes his mind and tells me to "follow your bliss," I'm not sure what I'll do. My options, as I see them, are:

(a) Accept myself for who I am. This would be the smart choice, but knowing myself as I do, this may be unrealistic.

(b) Have my wrinkles "disappeared" (as if they were mob informants).

(c) Pack up the family and hit the road in search of a safe haven where cosmetic-procedure abstainers can live in (delusional) peace. Or

(d) File a class-action suit on behalf of the cosmetic underclass, claiming we're the victims of unfair competition. We'll probably lose, but maybe we can tie the matter up in court long enough for our friends' wrinkles to come back, if only temporarily.

2.

Older Women, Younger Shirts

You can wear shorts in your fifties and impress your peer group no end. But that doesn't mean you don't look 50; it just means you look 50 in a new way.
—*SUNDAY TIMES* (OF LONDON)

The mall has become a wasteland. Too old for H&M, too young for J. Jill, I wander its wilderness. Shuffling empty-handed from store to store, I pass other forlorn souls dressed, like me, in clothing from seasons long past, desperate to buy something current but unable to find a single garment capable of achieving a look that says, "I still care—don't count me out—but I'm not delusional." Oh, to sashay in a mini without looking like I'm trying too hard. My heart aches for sundresses and barely-there tops. I'm sitting shivah for Anthropologie, mourning the loss of J. Crew. Entire sections of the Gap are dead to me. At Urban Outfitters, I rush to tell the fresh-faced sales-child I'm not shopping for myself before she revs up a snide remark. But darn it, I won't go gentle into the dark night of Talbots sensible everything. I'm raging against Chico's wearable art and boring Coldwater Creek. Eileen Fisher's drapey layers will be the final nail in my coffin.

How I yearn for the long-lost days when the hunt for new clothes was exhilarating, when each outfit held at least the promise of transformation. I'd hit the stores with a persona in mind—foreign correspondent, preppie, hippie, hottie. Clothing was a costume, and shopping for my character was fun. I bought what I liked—outfits that said smart, outdoorsy, sexy—with fit and price the only considerations. But now, alas, a single uptight question rules every purchase: Is it *appropriate*?

Can I tell you how I've come to resent that word, with its prissy rules and judgmental ways? Appropriate is the Miss Congeniality of attributes. It's not "hot" or "great" or even "interesting." It's the slog-along, practical "what's best for you at this stage, dear." Just kill me now, before I go to one more event looking pleasant but forgettable, a brunette in not just sensible shoes but a sensible skirt and top, too. One of my friends insists appropriate is a "step up" from "flattering," which she sees as code for "This is passable, considering what you're working with," but I disagree. It's death by monotony.

Where once my mother's voice (in my head) accompanied me on shopping trips, advising against light-colored suede ("very expensive to clean") or overclingy skirts ("You don't want to look cheap"), it's now my inner critic, the one who speaks for society, that has a bullhorn: "Don't show your knees," it commands. "A jean jacket is harsh near the face." "Pink looks little-girlish." I know the fashion police won't literally confront me if I step out of line. Unsuitable clothing choices aren't governed by the same rules that pertain to cell phone use. But even so, the citizen militia—many of them women in the same boat—are always on guard, ready to hiss their harsh verdict: "Look at her—with the too-long hair, the skintight jeans, the cowboy boots, the wrinkly cleavage—she's *desperate*." I myself have thrown such stones.

But anyone, even the most cautious, can commit a fashion felony. Sometimes a saleswoman—perhaps ignorant, perhaps more concerned with her commission than your dignity—gives bad advice. Or maybe a friend has started Dressing Under the Influence (DUI) of her teenage daughter, and you figure, hey, why can't I go a little more youthful, too? Or the combination of a looming party and an empty closet throws you into a mentally unstable, easily suggestible state in which your credit cards should be frozen for your protection. I was in precisely such a vulnerable pre-event condition when I found myself in a boutique whose rightful clientele are people born the year I graduated from college. "That top is ah-*door*-able," the owner gushed when she saw me sneaking a peek at a white blouse with puffy short sleeves, a ruffled front, and a collar best described as "sweet." It was indeed the Dakota Fanning of garments, but that was precisely the problem. Its own adorability would throw my lack of youthful perkiness into greater relief. Wouldn't I be better off with a top admired for its handsomeness?

"Don't be silly," the owner said. "The sleeves aren't too young?" I asked. "No," she countered, eager to move the merchandise. "Your arms are still good."

Still.

Here I was, the mother of two, fertility worries thankfully behind me, trapped in a dressing room, deafened by the ticking of my arms' biological clock. Is there no part of the body that won't desert you? Which organ or limb would be next? My legs? Probably—my knees are already halfway out the door. I started to panic. I could sense the owner hovering on the other side of the velvet drapes. "What are we thinking about the shirt?" she asked. Did she want the truth? That on a seemingly pleasant Thursday afternoon the innocuous little white blouse triggered a minor crisis? That sometimes I'm so insecure about my age that a piece of *clothing* can make me feel sad? That In My Day, I wore sundresses and tank tops and tooled around in flip-flops without worrying about my feet, and my gosh they're not kidding when they say "life is not a dress rehearsal" and it all goes so fast and—"I'll take it," I said.

My credit card was still in my physical custody—I was just handing it over—when I began to regret my purchase. I knew I was making a mistake, yet I was powerless to pull back. "Returns are for merchandise credit only," she said. I nodded sadly. We both knew that other than the blouse, which itself was wrong, there was not a single thing in the entire store a woman my age could "get away with." Even the coin purses were too young.

Dressing for the party a few hours later, trying to imagine what the hostess, a high-profile style editor, would think of my new purchase, I started in on Ken. "Is this shirt too young for me?" "No, you always look great." As any wife knows, a husband's first response to this question is just a starting point in the discussion, not the final word. The conversation isn't officially over until you've tricked him into inadvertently saying something that can be taken as an offense. "The sleeves aren't too cutesy?" "Not at all." "Are the ruffles too much?" "No, they're fine." I had him on the ropes. "Just *fine*?" He looked up from his computer and considered not just the shirt, but my flared orange skirt. "Okay," he said, "you look like you could be in a musical." If you knew Ken, you'd understand he wasn't trying to be mean or to make a bitchy remark, like one of those snarky on-air fashion commentators. He meant what he said literally. He was struggling to label my look. And I had to hand it to him. He, a man who could not tell you whether round-toed shoes are in or out for spring, had pinpointed an issue that had escaped my imagination. I'd been so worried about being "mutton dressed as lamb," to use the horrible British expression, that I'd overlooked a more egregious problem: I appeared as if I might break into song. And I know you'll believe me when I say that "middle-aged woman in a community theater production" is not the look I was after. But between the flouncy shirt and the flamenco-inspired skirt, I could see his point. Even so, I'd hoped I had more of a sexy Spanish look going. "You don't think Penélope Cruz might have worn this in *Volver?*" I suggested. He shook his head. "Rita Moreno in *West Side Story.*"

Although research on the psychology of dressing is woefully slim, several U.K. academics have not only looked at women's "relationships" with their clothing but also validated the very concept. Writing in the *Journal of Gender Studies* in 2000, Ali Guy and Maura Banim observed that women have a "dynamic relationship with their clothes that can be grouped around three co-existing views of self; 'The woman I want to be,' 'The woman I fear I could be' and 'The woman I am most of the time.'"

And I'll add: the woman who wants something new to wear. Like a lot of my sartorially adrift contemporaries, I wonder why the clothing industry isn't dying to cater to a group that's so eager to acquire. Get middle-aged women started on the subject of fashion, and the mournful lack of options is a constant refrain. "I have nothing to wear" has been replaced with something even worse: "There's nothing to buy." Our credit cards are ready, but they remain unswiped. Curious as to how retailers could have overlooked an enormous opportunity, I called Mintel International Group, a market research firm, and asked to speak with an analyst. Instead an assistant emailed me a report that pretty much answered my question. Ladies, guess who's being blamed for the lack of stores catering to the thirty-five-plus market? That's right: we are—the victims. Almost one fourth of the women in Dove's 2006 "Beauty Comes of Age" survey said they resist shopping because of age-related discomfort; we stay away because we're made to feel awkward and now it's our fault?

But let's get to Mintel's report: "Traditionally, the women's clothing market has focused a great deal on younger consumers," it began. Okay, thank you, but we already know this. That's the *problem*. The dearth of stores called "Forever 51" is sort of a tip-off. "Consumer data suggest reasons why this might be so," the report continues. "While women 18–24 are not more likely than all women to have shopped for clothes/accessories in the past year (89% vs. 88% of the total), they are more likely to have bought a greater variety of clothing (5.01 types vs. 4.30 types)." Gee, I wonder why. Do you think it has something to do with the fact that society so limits the styles older women can wear that entire regions of the body must be covered, as if for religious purposes?

This younger group, the report tells us, "is more receptive to trends, which suggests higher rates of wardrobe turnover. Indeed, 18% of those 18–24 'agree a lot' with the statement: 'I like to experiment with new styles' (7 points higher than average). And, some 11% 'agree a lot' with 'every season I buy the latest fashions' (6 points higher)." Mintel people, if you're reading this: I'm in my mid-forties, and I "agree a lot" with the statement: "Every season I wear the same thing I wore last season, and if I have to face that pair of black velvet pants one more time, I won't be able to attend any more parties."

So let me see if I've got this right: No one will open a store to sell me clothes because I don't shop enough, but I can't shop because there are no stores for me. I'm sorry, really I am, that I'm not buying the "latest" fashions, it's just that it's hard when the only pants I can find are obscene, and the dresses make me look pregnant (although now that I think about it, that would suggest youth, at least from a distance).

Let's keep reading: "The 45+ market needs comfortable, yet sophisticated clothing. Both the styles and the fabric should last, as this group leans toward conservative styles and has a tendency to 'make their clothing last.'" Excuse me, but it's not a "tendency"—it's desperation. I'd love to discard clothes simply because they're last season's, but I hold on for dear life to everything I have for fear I'll never be able to replace it and then I'll end up with literally nothing in my closet (as opposed to the "nothing" that denotes a closet full of unacceptable garments; like bimonthly, *nothing* can mean two completely different things). I don't want a top with a strange neckline, detail, or hood, or one that's ridiculously long or short (a rib-cage-grazing sweatshirt?), or any article of clothing that bears no resemblance to the human shape.

"While many Boomers are able and willing to spend on items they want, many are more cautious and thrifty than the general adult population." Why? Because we've spent the past few decades getting burned. We have fashion baggage. We remember the poison purchases of yesteryear. Pronouncements such as "Metallic puce is the new black!" and "Capris are the It pant of the season!" ring in our ears. Perhaps ours is a caution born of experience.

And guess what else? We're being punished because we're unwilling to travel half a day to get what we need. "Convenient location of retail stores is also very important to Boomers, with nearly 60% of Boomers responding that they only shop at stores located near their homes." Forgive me if I've got grocery shopping to do and dinner to make and homework to monitor and an article to write and a contractor to nag and laundry to fold and presents to wrap and holiday cards to address.

To be fair, the industry does make periodic stabs at trying to get our money, although it seems baffled about how to go about it. As *BusinessWeek* asked in April of 2007: "What do 35-year-old women want?" How about clothing we can wear? The story reported that Bloomingdale's is going after an "elusive" demographic other retailers tried and failed to win. It just figures, doesn't it? We're playing hard to get, and it's for something we *want.* "Gymboree Corp., known for its children's clothing, shuttered Janeville, its brand for women in their mid-30s and older," *BusinessWeek* wrote. "Soon after, Gap Inc. announced it would close its Forth & Towne division, which targeted a similar shopper."

I never went anywhere near a Forth & Towne. I'm sure I would have found something I liked—I heard the pants fit nicely—but I was afraid that I'd actually buy something, be complimented on it at work, and then age shame would force me to lie about its provenance. Being a known Forth & Towne shopper would be like wearing your AARP membership card on your sleeve. As one commentator wrote in an online forum about the *BusinessWeek* article: "Transitioning from shopping in the young women's section to a section targeted at slightly older women can be a very tangible sign of age for many women (conjuring a certain 'can you believe what kids these days are wearing?' sort of dowdiness)."

I thought back to when I was a child in the 1960s, a time when little girls wanted to dress like their mothers but were often forbidden from wearing styles that were "too old" for them. Now mothers are raiding their tweens' closets—a strange state of affairs captured by a *New Yorker* cartoon showing a mother poking her head into her daughter's room. "Can Mommy borrow your baby-blue pinafore tonight, sweetie?" she asks. How did we get to a place where almost all females— from age eight to eighty—dress alike? It turns out that cultural forces set in motion after World War II, when teens first got spending power, and with it, market clout, are responsible for postmenopausal women shopping at Express.

Social historian Lynne Luciano Loeb looked back to the mid-1960s, when, "along with the phraseology of 'Don't trust anyone over thirty,' came the youth quake, and the belief that immaturity is superior to maturity. The lifestyles of college-age [people] really came to the forefront then," she said. "Young people became very visible and very appealing and very contemptuous of the older generation—and I mean people in their thirties and forties. Youth became the desirable age. You began seeing a blurring of aging lines as older people strive to 'age down' rather than younger people trying to 'age up.'"

Okay, so we know *why* we have the problem, but that still doesn't help us find an outfit.

For advice on that, I turned to Simon Doonan, the creative director of Barneys New York and author of the 2008 *Eccentric Glamour: Creating an Insanely More Fabulous You.* Considering that the very act of entering one of his stores, with their trendy clothes and youthful employees, has set off an incalculable number of age-related wardrobe meltdowns, I was surprised by his counsel: "I think the whole idea of growing old gracefully is absurd. Age should give you carte blanche to do whatever the hell you want. Our culture is so youth-centered. The tendency is to be overly judgmental about older people and underly judgmental about younger people. People will castigate some middle-aged woman for dressing in a fast, cheeky way, but there's got to be some payoff [for getting older]. In our culture, once people get over forty-five they are completely ignored."

His remark about the invisibility of the over-forty-five was something I'd heard quite often (give or take a few years). And it got me wondering: Just *who* is doing all this ignoring? If it's the youth, why do we invest them with such power? And if it's us, why are we disregarding our contemporaries? But those weren't questions for Simon, and when you have an influential style guru on the line you don't interrupt him. "One person's idea of appropriate is another person's idea of boring," he continued.

"There's no such thing as a faux pas once you get older," he concluded. "If a middle-aged woman feels good in butt-crack jeans, why shouldn't she have fun?"

Simon's comments made me feel so empowered I almost put on my frilly white shirt—almost. But then I thought about something Andrea Linett, the creative director of *Lucky* magazine, told me. "Certain people get away with things and certain people don't." I knew which category I was in. "If Cher was wearing something 'appropriate,' she'd look like she's trying too hard. You have to find your natural balance and stay with it." So true, and yet so impossible. "It's easier said than done," she acknowledged. "But if you feel like you're wearing a costume, then you probably look like you're wearing a costume."

And about to break out singing "I Want to Live in America."

I was trying to figure out how to become one of those lucky souls who can "get away" with something (such as cowboy boots paired with a thigh-grazing dress) when celebrity stylist and TV personality Phillip Bloch returned my call. Fresh off an "exhausting" shoot with Michael Jackson, he offered advice that seemed a bit safer than Simon's: "The most important thing is knowing your body type and what works on your body," he explained. "And you have to be attuned to what your life is now. Are you a mom? Are you working? Are you dressing appropriately for what you do?" Well, if what I do is walk around looking schleppy, then yes! I am dressed perfectly. "Age," he added, "is really how you present yourself, and how people see you and not the number."

Actually, age can be a plus! At least according to the "Glam Gals" behind the "Fabulous After 40" website. "We've coined 'age-mazing' instead of 'age-appropriate,'" JoJami Tyler told me. "That means women don't necessarily want to look twentysomething, nor like their grandmothers. They want to look like they haven't given up on themselves. But we get stuck in a rut."

Never mind that I *would* like to look twentysomething, I asked Tyler how to achieve this age-mazing look. Add a single youthful element to an outfit, she said. Pair conservative jeans with a fun top. "And we have to start wearing better-quality clothes," she insisted. "We've been so educated and brainwashed that we have to buy on sale. We all want that little sale fix or hit and we have all these cheapie pieces in our wardrobe. This is just making you look bad. Get your budget and find that gorgeous piece."

The experts make shopping sound so straightforward, don't they? I read their advice in the magazines or see them on TV and every single time I think, Oh yes, of course, just a few basic pieces snazzed up with accessories! Then I venture back into the stores and get intimidated all over again. "If only we had someone to blame," a friend said after returning empty-handed from yet another shopping trip. "They should be called 'looking' trips," she noted. We cast around for a perpetrator and hit on an entire class of villains: the young people. Why are they at fault, they who don't even care about us, don't even see us? Because they're bleaching their teeth at twenty and doing preventative sunscreening and cosmetic work, which means they'll never look old, an effect that will age us even further as the apparent disparity in our ages grows. And as if that isn't enough, one of the most upsetting fashion stories I read recently wasn't about a style that's too young for me, but rather one that, theoretically, is made specifically *for* me. In London, twentysomethings are wearing middle-aged clothing styles, as if to prove it's not the dresses, but the dresser, that ruins the look.

The headline in the British paper the *Observer* played on the infamous "mutton dressed as lamb" phrase to ask: "Are you lamb dressed as mutton? Dressing 20 years too old? Cool! Flash, trash and flesh are over—demure knits and kitten heels are hot." Except, of course, for people whose only options *are* demure knits and kitten heels. If you're middle-aged, the article pointed out, "middle-aged chic" is not for you. "You'll find this out in your own good time, but I'd like to spare you some fashion pain if at all poss, so listen up. The problem with [middle-aged chic] is that a) it's not very sexy, so you won't want to attempt it if you're on the pull in any way, shape or form; and b) ironically enough, it's very hard to do if you actually are middle aged. You'll just look frumpy. Don't do it passed [*sic*] thirty-eight."

Okay, I give up. Not only can't we dress young, we can't dress our age. No wonder so many middle-aged women start collecting patchwork jackets made from retired saris and sporting enormous pins. But be careful. Accessories that serve as conversation pieces, along with turtlenecks out of season, are the red flags of an AWOL wardrobe.

And yet, as difficult as finding an appropriate little black dress remains, I've come to learn that middle-aged women aren't the only ones stressing about the age-appropriate issue. Not long after the puffy-sleeved shirt incident, I was browsing the Internet with my sons looking for a towel for my kindergartner to use at school at naptime. We checked out the many superhero options, and finally he decided he liked Buzz Lightyear the best. "Should I order it?" I asked. "No," he said sadly. "The kids will think it's babyish."

And so it begins.

3.

Pore, Pore, Pitiful Me

Nature gives you the face you have at 20.
It is up to you to merit the face
you have at 50.
—COCO CHANEL

I'm no dermatologist. I don't even know what copper peptides do. But I had an epiphany while applying my morning dose of face cream: if using this stuff *twice* a day, as instructed, diminishes the appearance of fine lines by 16 percent—or 23 percent or whatever they have the cheek to claim—then slathering it on *hourly* would work miracles, no?

That was the logic behind my decision to binge on a tub of Dr. Patricia Wexler's Skin Regenerating Serum. I'd gotten it as a freebie from the fashion editor at work, and after reading that it "visibly repairs and improves skin inside and out" and "reverses the lines, sink and sag," it was obvious that only a fool would use it sparingly. My plan was to put away the whole container before my early-afternoon column deadline. "How does my face look?" I asked the fashion editor halfway through my bender. We're friends, but I got the sense she was regretting her generosity. "Don't touch my keyboard," she said, sashaying to a photo shoot.

As if I'd have time. Between the serum application, finger cleansing, and mirror visits, my schedule was packed. "Everything . . . okay?" the features editor asked after my fourth trip to the ladies' room. Was it? Maybe the serum had addled my mind, but I swear I detected a waxy buildup, the kind Brand X tables suffer from in Lemon Pledge commercials. I stared at my reflection, but for the life of me, I couldn't recall what my face had looked like when it left for work that morning. Uncertain of my results—but sure I was on to *something,* I called the American Academy of Dermatology seeking an expert opinion. The PR person referred me to Dr. Alexa Kimball, the director of a research unit at the world-renowned Massachusetts General Hospital. It's embarrassing to ask a respected clinical investigator such a superficial question, but I knew I couldn't let self-consciousness stop me. What if I'd discovered a breakthrough application schedule that had—somehow—escaped every vice president of marketing in the multibillion-dollar global beauty industry? I was pondering my Nobel ceremony outfit—scratch that, my *Oprah* outfit—when Dr. Kimball came on the line. "Dr. Kimball," I began. She interrupted me. "Beth, it's me, Alexa. I met you at the——'s party last week." Oh right, of course, Alexa *Kimball,* the dermatologist I'd been talking to while I wolfed down shrimp. (A friend who entertains frequently once observed that you see a different side of people when you put out shrimp, and I've found it to be one of the truest things I've ever heard.) As I feared, it turns out that after a certain point, not only does your face derive no additional benefit from extracurricular applications but it could also become irritated. A single application of any given skin cream usually delivers about 75 or 80 percent of the goods, Dr. Kimball explained, and then the returns start diminishing. At some point you cross the line from merely wasting time and money to potentially causing a problem that necessitates yet another product.

I had been planning to ask Dr. Kimball about a second scheme I'd concocted, in which you use a different product every hour, allowing you to pack in glycolic acid, antioxidants, vitamins C and E, soy, and those baffling copper peptides all in one day, but I'd gleaned an important if disappointing take-home message from her first response: You can't beat the system. Fighting wrinkles is like gambling; the house always wins.

Saddened, I tried to hustle Dr. Kimball off the phone, but the doctor wanted something publicized, and because she hadn't mocked my attempts at lay dermatology—and also because she's one of the few dermatologists around not pushing her own skin care line—I felt she deserved a forum. "Please, please, please," she begged, "debunk the water myth. It's ridiculous. All the beauty magazines say you need to drink six to eight glasses a day to keep your skin hydrated. There is no evidence that it goes to your face. Blood, water, and salt move in very specific ways in the body. [The water] is mostly going into your bloodstream and being peed out by the kidneys."

Only in cases of extreme dehydration, she said, would your face be affected. Like if you were crawling through the desert on all fours with the sun beating down, and you were so parched you couldn't speak— then maybe the situation would take its toll on your skin. But at that point, your appearance would be the last thing on your mind. Well, probably. Actually maybe not. You never know when you're going to be rescued by a search team with CNN in tow.

I was about to put down the huge sports bottle from which I'd been dutifully (pointlessly?) sipping, but water's gotten such consistently great buzz I figured I should get a second opinion. I called Dr. Nicholas Perricone, a dermatologist with not only his own skin care line but also a bunch of bestselling antiwrinkle books. Water is his thing. "You don't get thirsty until you're 3 percent dehydrated," he warned, "and when you're even slightly dehydrated it increases inflammation." Inflammation is the "bad guy" that leads to, among other problems, "rapid aging and wrinkles," he told me. Critics have accused him of making claims just to sell books, but as Renée Zellweger would say, he had me at "rapid aging."

I took a big long gulp of Poland Spring and wondered whether water is the world's oldest facial cosmetic, or if I should stick to the Olay. Either way, one thing is for sure: "Every system in your body depends on water. Water flushes toxins out of vital organs, carries nutrients to your cells and provides a moist environment for ear, nose and throat tissues." That's from the website of the Mayo Clinic. And this is from every chicken-soup-pushing Jewish grandmother I've ever known: "It couldn't hurt."

As for my skin care plans, I was back to my usual M.O.: Rush out and buy the latest must-have cream.

Smear it on and look in the mirror for results. Notice no difference. Toss it in the medicine cabinet and begin the search for new miracle product. Repeat. If you were to try to guess my goal from observing my behavior, you could be forgiven for thinking my objective was to waste as much money and packaging as possible—to contribute my part to global warming, one plastic tube at a time. "Maybe you should stick to a product for a while and see what happens," Ken suggested. For space reasons his shaving supplies had been moved to the kids' bathroom, so I suspected his advice was motivated less by dermatological wisdom than by turf issues, but even so he was probably right. "Don't be ridiculous," I said.

I knew my behavior wasn't productive, but I didn't realize just how absurd my expectations were until I heard an Estée Lauder executive discussing the challenge of the impatient consumer. If she doesn't see results almost immediately, Dr. Daniel Maes said during a panel discussion at the Health & Beauty America convention, she'll abandon the product. Give up almost immediately. I found myself snickering, until I realized he was describing me. I thought we consumers were the only ones with a problem, but the skin care makers face a challenge, too: antiwrinkle technologies can take weeks to work (if indeed they do work), but in an age of instant gratification, no one wants to wait.

What's a poor global corporation to do? Estée Lauder, among other companies, adds light-scattering components to some antiwrinkle products, thereby reducing the appearance of imperfections while the technology gets to work on the actual imperfections. The aim is to retain the customer during the difficult you-gotta-believe phase. Maes used terms like "optical technologies" and "polymers" to describe the additives, but I thought of them as the glass of wine the restaurant owner sends over to keep you happy until your table—finally—becomes available.

I can't remember what keywords I gave Google to come up with the name of David Miller, but the moment I got him on the line, it was obvious I'd found a man with an answer to Life's Big Question. What is the real meaning of one of the most common marketing lines of our times: "reduces the *appearance* of fine lines"?

Dr. Miller is the president of CuDerm Corp., a Dallas-based laboratory that measures pore size and wrinkle depth for major cosmetic companies, and he spends his days analyzing negative replica masks of subjects' faces. In his world, lines and wrinkles look like mountain ridges, and pores like Hershey's Kisses.

But of course they're nowhere near that big. When Miller told me the average fine line is less than one-tenth of a millimeter deep, I almost went into shock. We've built a multibillion-dollar industry fighting an enemy thinner than a strand of hair.

Dr. Miller is a man of science, with a doctorate in physical chemistry, but he takes a lighthearted approach to his work. In his office he keeps a quote from Ava Gardner: "Let me read it to you," he said. "'Whatever wrinkles I got, I enjoyed getting them.'" He chuckled. Like a detective with an appreciation for his quarry, Miller *likes* wrinkles. "They're a sign of life in your body," he said. "If we eliminate them, there goes character down the drain. We don't want to look like dolls or mannequins."

"Speak for yourself," I said.

"Other people's wrinkles earn me money," he said.

I'd always assumed that the "appearance" claim was a dodge that allowed cosmetics makers to trick consumers into thinking significant clinical results had been achieved when in fact they hadn't. The Food and Drug Administration regulates substances that change the structure of the skin, but products that merely assert to alter the "appearance" of imperfections are allowed to operate without FDA meddling. (For fun reading, visit the agency's website, www.fda.gov, and check out the warning letter section. On the day I clicked, I found a letter to the maker of the seductive LiftFusion, a cream that claims to be the first "topical-injectable alternative to doctor-administered anti-wrinkle injections." The firm was spanked for claiming that its product was "proven more effective than Botox® in a clinical study" and "helps reduce existing wrinkles AND boost collagen to promote skin's natural defenses against new ones.")

But as far as the "appearance" word goes, guess what? It's not always a sign of duplicity. "There is truth in the appearance claim," Miller informed me. "There are plenty of ways to change the appearance of a wrinkle without making it disappear."

One way to achieve this miracle is to change the way light bounces off the face. Yes, the wrinkles still exist, but if you're using cosmetics with light-throwing minerals, they're not as visible. "The eye of the beholder misses some of the wrinkles," Miller said.

How? An MIT professor once told me to think of a wrinkle as a black hole; any light that comes close bounces in and gets absorbed. But with the right kind of reflective powder, the light can bounce right back out again, thereby making the furrow more similar in appearance to the skin around it.

The only drawback is that in order to get the light-bouncing benefits, you have to be wearing the product. Which means that if a fire breaks out in your house in the middle of the night, the first thing you should do, before grabbing your new Coach bag or weighing yourself, is apply a light-scattering foundation.

"What the appearance claim is really saying," Miller said, "is we didn't necessarily measure the wrinkles' depth or frequency, but we took a bunch of pictures and showed them to experts and they said the wrinkles looked diminished."

The bottom line? In skin care, as in politics, appearances matter.

And, as Miller noted, "that includes the appearance of the jar. The high-end companies spend a lot of money on packaging. One of my colleagues says that if you could figure out a nice way to package lard, it would make a great moisturizer."

We were about to get off the phone, but one question was still nagging at me. What baseline do the makers of cosmetics creams use for comparison? Will I see a reduction in fine lines if I switch from my product to theirs, or do I need to be in a really bad place, skin-wise, to get the promised benefits? Here's where things get interesting. In many studies, subjects undergo a so-called washout period, during which they use no moisturizer at all—only soap and water. Miller told me that this is a "valid scientific approach for 'leveling the playing field,' so to speak," but, he added, "it can lead to improvements measured in the clinical study that may not be duplicated in the real world. Skin, like life, is complicated."

Meanwhile, all this talk about the way light hits the face made me think about how many times I'd been in a conference room or a restaurant with a wall of windows and wondered, from an appearance perspective, if I'd be better off sitting with my back or my face to the light source. I put the question to the scion of the prominent Bachrach photography studio, Robert Bachrach, a man who's made portraits of Ronald Reagan, Meryl Streep, and Dizzie Gillespie, among others. "Do you mean where should you sit to have your picture taken?" he asked. "No, where should I sit so I look better when I'm out and about."

"That's a good question," he said. "If the window is facing north, that light is soft light, so in that case you want to be facing the window." However, if the window is facing south, you want the sun behind you, so have it to your back. Even if it means you have to wrestle your companion for the more advantageous seat. If you don't have a good sense of direction, you may want to carry a compass. Just pretend it's a compact when you pull it out.

The fact that January 2007 didn't go down as the month that changed everything says all we need to know about the power of marketing—and hope. That's when *Consumer Reports* published its study showing that "on average these [over-the-counter skin creams] made little difference in the skin's appearance, and there's no correlation between price and effectiveness."

Little difference in the skin's appearance? We've got half the population consumed with products that do essentially nothing? Can someone do an intervention, please?

But wait, that was just the beginning. The magazine also reported that "*CR*'s tests found no relationship between the types of active ingredients in the products and their overall performance." I put down the report and caught my breath. This was even harder than learning that one of the coauthors of *The Rules: Time-Tested Secrets for Capturing the Heart of Mr. Right* was getting divorced. Where do I go from here? I wondered.

To be fair, the skin care products didn't do literally nothing. "In *CR*'s tests, the top-rated products did smooth out some fine lines and wrinkles after 12 weeks. But even the best performers reduced the average depth of wrinkles by less than 10 percent, a magnitude of change that was barely visible to the naked eye."

Barely visible to the naked eye. All this time and effort to achieve results that you'd need a microscope to detect.

The best of the lot, *CR* reported, was Olay Regenerist, which is available in drugstores for about $19 apiece for the "enhancing lotion," "perfecting cream," and "regenerating serum" combination recommended by the company. At $176, "Lancôme Paris Rénergie" performed nearly as well"—well, yippee! Meanwhile, the most costly product tested, La Prairie Cellular ($335 for an ounce of day cream and 1.7 ounces of night cream), was "among the least effective."

I figured La Prairie would be too embarrassed to show its face after that assessment, and kind of curious, I hustled over to Neiman Marcus expecting to see the counter dark. But it was bustling. I hovered around a bit. "Can I help you?" the saleslady asked. I picked up a tester of the Cellular Intensive Anti-Wrinkle & Anti-Spot Cream. "Does this stuff work?" I asked in as judgment-free a voice as possible. "It's been doing *fabulous* for us," she said. Sure, it helps the store, but what about *me*? I tried again. "Does it work on, you know, the skin?" She took out a little spatula and spread some on my hand. "It literally interferes with cells losing moisture," she said. Then she used what I think of as "the nurse's 'we,'" as in, "How are we feeling today?" "As we get older our cells get flatter. This plumps them up."

"Thanks," I said, heading away from the counter. "I'll give it some thought." "I'm——if you need anything," she said. Like what—to be suckered in? I'll make sure to ask for you the next time I want to make a faith-based purchase.

Considering that no one I knew changed her behavior based on the *Consumer Reports* study, I thought maybe it was a figment of my wrinkle-obsessed imagination, but I found a similarly negative article in Harvard Medical School's *HEALTHbeat* newsletter (published in the spring of 2006). "No moisturizer can make wrinkles disappear or prevent new ones from forming, and none can stop the effects of gravity or exposure to sunlight," *HEALTHbeat* reported. "There's no proof that vitamins or antioxidants applied directly to the skin do much at all.

"Nor is it known whether they remain active long enough to prevent cell damage, promote new collagen production, or confer other benefits," the newsletter continued. "Vitamin C [ascorbic acid], for example, quickly loses potency when exposed to the air. So, it's unlikely that vitamin C in skin creams offers much benefit. Vitamin E is believed to improve the appearance of scars and help speed wound-healing. But there's no evidence that it does. And in some people, topical vitamin E causes allergic reactions."

I wondered if I should run to the closest mall, where my sisters were laying down all sorts of good money, and yell "Fire."

You know, these studies are almost enough to make me think that as a society we should redefine success. Obviously we enjoy the purchasing portion of the anti-wrinkle fight; so let's keep doing that as usual and just change the goal. Considering that skin worsens by the day, maybe simply holding the line should constitute "progress." That sounds pessimistic, but wouldn't you be thrilled to look like you do today at eighty-five?

And yet, the news from Harvard wasn't *all* bad. A few things do work.

- "Aging skin often looks rough and sallow because it doesn't slough off dead surface skin cells as easily as younger skin," the newsletter said, explaining that two chemical exfoliants—alpha hydroxy acids and beta hydroxy acids—are believed to renew the skin more effectively than many scrubs, masks, soaps, toners, or abrasive cloths.

- And: "Vitamins don't generally reduce wrinkles, with the exception of the topical vitamin A-based drugs called *retinoids.* Tretinoin, marketed as Retin-A and Renova, is the most common retinoid used in skin care. Introduced in the 1970s as an acne treatment, tretinoin demonstrated an ability to speed the turnover of superficial skin cells."

I made a mental note to myself to exfoliate with an alpha or beta hydroxy acid, and to get myself a prescription for Renova, stat, if it wouldn't break the bank. I called my insurer to see if vanity visits to the dermatologist are covered. Tension twisted my gut, but oh, happy day. (Or happy*ish* day. It turned out that while my appointment required only a co-pay, any prescription I filled would be out-of-pocket.) A few weeks later I was sitting in a doctor's office, my cheeks flushed with anticipation. I hadn't looked so naturally rosy in years. "Have you noticed a change in any moles?" the dermatologist asked. I had not. "Any skin growths that concern you?" There were none. "Any change in anything?" No. The issue hung in the air: Why was I there? "Uh, I'd like some Renova." I felt like an addict trying to score prescription-strength painkillers.

She took my face in her hands and examined it. I had come specifically for an antiaging product, but even so, I was hoping she'd say I didn't need it. If you surround yourself with the right kind of friends/partners/sycophants, you can have a wrinkle that would show up as Mount Everest in Dr. Miller's laboratory and everyone will swear she doesn't see it.

"You're a good candidate for it," the doctor said. "You've got fine lines and signs of sun damage." She pulled out her prescription pad, asked me what size tube of Renova I wanted, and instructed me to use it once a day, or every other day, or every three days if I noticed irritation. She obviously didn't know who she was dealing with. Finally! After all these years spent wandering in the wilderness, I was poised to turn back time. But despite Vitamin A's excellent reputation, after all I'd read about products making only infinitesimal differences, I was curious to see for myself if even the vaunted Renova could achieve detectable improvements. I decided to conduct a split-face study of my own, similar to the ones performed by Dr. Miller's lab. I would apply Renova to one half of my face daily, and the other half would get some over-the-counter cream. I'm sure Dr. Miller would have sent me one of his rubbery-mask kits so I could measure my results in a scientifically rigorous way, but if I couldn't detect improvement in non-laboratory conditions, what difference would it make anyway? If a wrinkle disappears in the forest. . . .

I was about to get started, but standing there in the bathroom, with the tube open, a pea-size dot on my finger, I realized I faced a huge research quandary. Which side of my face should enjoy the Renova? I imagined the treated side living the life of a twenty-something, getting carded at bars, being whistled at on the street, wearing flip-flops in winter, while the control side held menus at arm's length so she could read the type.

Left or right? I hadn't been expecting to play God.

The only criteria I could think of was that when we were in the car Ken was on my left, so that side might be more important, although I usually turn to talk to him, so, oh, who knows? I made a snap decision. The left side would be the beneficiary. But there was no way I was using a placebo on the control side. At my age, I'm not sacrificing *anything* for science. I went with some Meokine Intensive Dermo-Crease Reducing Corrective Wrinkle Care cream I'd picked up at CVS. It sounded excellent—"dermo-crease reducing!" who even knew such a phrase existed— but even so, I was already pitying the right side of my face, poised, as it was, to look like an old lady by comparison. Until I read the package inserts for both creams, which is when I began to worry about the Renova side.

While the Meokine promised precisely the kind of miracle I sought—it "smoothes skin creases and helps erase wrinkles"—Renova basically promised to do nothing. "RENOVA DOES NOT ELIMINATE WRINKLES, REPAIR SUN-DAMAGED SKIN, REVERSE PHOTO-AGING, OR RESTORE MORE YOUTHFUL OR YOUNGER SKIN," the package insert read in boldfaced capital letters.

For this I paid $160 of my own money?

"Just ignore it," my friend advised. "They have to say that."

"Really? Why? Because it's true?" "Don't be so negative," she said. "Your skin will pick up on the bad vibe." She directed my attention to an article in the November 30, 2006, issue of the *New York Times*. "The thing about Retin-A," the Styles section headline read, "It works." That was enough for me. I didn't even need to read the whole story to learn about tretinoins' clinically proven ability to increase collagen production and smooth wrinkles and fade age spots; the headline alone had validated my skin care choice.

I was on the brink of starting my experiment when I realized I hadn't given any thought to ethical questions: What if the Renova side thrives while the other continues its downward march? Would it be morally right to carry on with the study? Or would I have to halt it instantly and begin emergency Renova applications?

(Or, as an alternative, wear a *Phantom of the Opera*–style mask covering the aging half?)

And ethics aside, I had an immediate, concrete problem. Because I couldn't draw a line to bisect my face, I worried that I'd inadvertently overlap the creams and end up with a flaming red stripe running down the middle of my face (although I guess that *would* draw attention away from the wrinkles). Conversely, if I was too conservative and left too much space between the creams, the middle of my face would be—I can barely stand the thought—productless. With these thoughts in mind, I began the experiment.

Giddy with anticipation, I could hardly wait to wake up the next morning and look in the mirror. And I wasn't the only eager antiaging beaver. With my father's fiftieth law school reunion looming, my mother began calling daily. She'd make small talk about the kids, a novel, world news, then get to her point: "Is it working?" Our conversations went on for weeks that way, until one day she called not to question, but to warn. Because Renova takes several months to work, she pointed out, it's possible that the right side of my face might never catch up. Forty years down the line it would still be months behind. I could go to my grave looking like a Picasso.

Reeling, I hung up and called Ken, hoping he'd dismiss her fear. "She may be right," he said. "You don't know what it's doing to your pigmentation."

"Someone call the Data Safety Monitoring Board," I cried out. "I'm halting the study right now."

The good news: I caught the situation in time and started smearing the cream over my whole face. If any Renova-related pigmentation changes *are* occurring, at least they'll be facewide. The bad news: I still have no way of knowing whether the stuff is working. I think my skin looks better, but since starting Renova I've also started using a tinted moisturizer that scatters light in a flattering way. So who knows? Maybe I don't look better, I just *appear* to.

4.

Post-Traumatic Tress Disorder

I could announce . . . that the world was
going to blow up in three hours and people
would be calling in about my hair!
—KATIE COURIC

I t begins innocently enough, as so many things do. Starting in their mid-thirties, women heed a silent call to lop off an inch or two of their hair. It's nothing drastic; the result is often met with compliments. But like the canary in the coal mine rasping its first nervous cough, this is a sign of badness wafting from a tunnel up ahead. Inevitably, some layering will follow, with additional trims to madame's coiffure, a bit more layering, then some bangs. Soon enough the hair starts its final ascent, passing the shoulders around age forty, and then the chin, and eventually settling at a wash-'n'-go ear-level helmet. Depending on the victim's hair color and political leanings, from behind she might be mistaken for Hillary Clinton or Laura Bush. We've witnessed the phenomenon on countless "women of a certain age," and the process is seemingly voluntary.

Unlike the "Farrah" or the "Rachel," this is a style that dares not speak its name. And despite near-total domination of its market segment, no one actually wants the coif. You don't settle into the stylist's chair, gaze in the mirror, and say, "I want a cut that will render me invisible to anyone under thirty, see what you can do," or "I'd like to highlight my crepey neck—give me the suburban helmet look." What you say is: "I want my hair to be fuller and have more bounce, *but I want to keep the length.*"

The stylist agrees, mentioning that the new cut will highlight your cheekbones or perhaps your eyes. "We'll do layers," she says. Never, oh never, is the word "shorter" uttered. "You want the gamine look!" she adds. Yes, you think, imagining that you'll walk out resembling Keira Knightley or Cameron Diaz. And so the shearing begins, and before you know it, you're being handed a mirror to check out your rear hair view. But wait, what's this? Where's Keira? Where's Cameron? They're nowhere to be found.

Instead, look which star has appeared: the fifth Golden Girl.

Even though you're present for the incremental shortening, you're never totally sure that it's happening until someone else points it out. You run into a former colleague and she says, "I like the short hair." "Short?" you say, "Actually, I'm due for a cut." Or maybe your child brings it up. I was walking my son to school one morning when we passed a young woman with long hair. She had the kind of simple, fuss-free straight hair that doesn't need layers or color or even a good blow-dry. For some reason my son noticed her and asked why I didn't have long hair. "I used to," I replied wistfully. "Why don't you now?" he wanted to know.

I used to think it was a DNA thing, that imprinted right there along with the "fight-or-flight" impulse was a biological directive that a woman over forty can't have hair beneath her shoulders. And indeed there's something to this, at least according to social scientists at Texas A & M University and the University of North Dakota, who did rigorous research on the matter and found a direct correlation between a woman's "reproductive status" (code word for "age") and the length of her hair. To put it in Freudian terms, as Wikipedia did, "psychoanalysts also see [long hair] in a sexual light, as a representation of the id's release from the suppression of the superego." And in Darwinian terms? "Scientists view long hair as playing a large part in any animal species' natural selection since hair length is frequently a sign of health," Wikipedia reports.

But even so, the received wisdom tells us that long hair is aging. It pulls the face down. That's what you're taught. And yet, celebrities—and women from sexier nations like Italy and Brazil (thank you, Sonia Braga)—manage to pull off flowing manes well into their fifties. Why can't we?

Maybe it's the hairdressers' fault. Popular wisdom knights the stylist as a girl's best friend, the one who takes her side against bad boyfriends and bosses. He's the soul mate/spirit lifter she parties with after splitting from her man. When the newly single Jennifer Aniston and Jessica Simpson hit the club scene with their hair gurus in tow, the executive editor of *In Style* magazine declared stylists "the new B.F." Gobbling up the stories and photos in the glossies, I coveted not just Aniston's and Simpson's locks, but the fawning attention they got from their hairdressers. My guy can't even remember on which side I part my hair, much less spend off-the-clock time with me.

I'm not saying stylists-to-the-schlubs don't care about their clients, but I fear boredom gets the better of them in the chair. I've yet to meet one who's content to dutifully trim my ends every eight weeks and leave it at that. You know the pattern: at first they hang on your every word like a lover. They *listen.* You want one quarter of an inch off? No problem, my *bella!* "I've found the One," you gush to friends. But no sooner have you renounced all others than monotony starts to set in—not on your end, but his—until he says the words you've heard so many times before: "Let's do something different today." You consent, of course, in a bid to save the relationship. Looking in the mirror, you praise his work, but in your heart you know you look like Nancy Pelosi.

Or maybe it's your friends who are to blame. How? I don't agree with the theory put forth in a 2006 issue of *Maxim* magazine that "despite always compliment-ing another woman's short haircut, she secretly cel-ebrates having one less competitor, since men prefer long hair." I think we're inadvertently doing each other in by being too nice. While no specific research has been done on women and compliments and short hair (except, apparently, by *Maxim*), a study that came out in 2007 on a phenomenon called "fat talk" found that women gain important mutual support from each other by complaining about their weight and receiving reas-surance. I called Denise Martz of Appalachian State University, a coauthor on the study, and asked her if the results were generalizable to the compliments we bestow when a friend shows up with a new—inevitably shorter—haircut. "Maybe as we age we learn to fish for compliments less and deliver them more, knowing that compliments, like any kind of social feedback, tend to be reciprocated," she said. In other words, I praise your short style and you in turn praise mine. It's a wonder any of us have any hair left at all. I ran my theory by Dr. Martz, and while she didn't disagree, she offered her own hypothesis: "This could be a practical issue. Short hair is easier. You get wiser as you age."

And I guess, to be fair, each woman owns at least some responsibility for her problems. Peer validation aside, we're the ones who keep rebooking with Suki or Fabio or whoever claims to be on the cutting edge of hip. Even as we complain, we tell ourselves "he wouldn't cut my hair this way unless it looked good," and "he understands me, I better not switch." And so you stay with the devil you know until your hair's shorter than your significant other's. Then and only then do you recognize the relationship has bottomed out. It's time to move on. And start the process again.

I was settling in for the unavoidable onset of the sensible-shoes hairstyle when an incredible opportunity presented itself: Frédéric Fekkai, the world-famous stylist to the stars, a man who gets $600 per cut, a guy who knows how to help a woman keep the length, was coming to Boston to celebrate the opening of a new upscale beauty boutique that sells his line of hair products. My *Boston Herald* editors and I had long been wondering just *how* good a haircut could be, and this seemed like the perfect opportunity to find out. You can bet that as a journalist, I don't make a salary that allows $600 haircuts (the tip alone would blow my budget), but my job as a columnist did have some perks, and one was about to come my way: if I was willing to report on the experience, Frédéric would do my hair for free.

But despite its $0 price tag, I wasn't sure the haircut assignment was such a good idea. Frédéric's offer was a onetime deal. Which meant that, at best, I would have this sassy, youthful haircut for six weeks, eight max, and then I'd be back to the Matron. Maybe it was better to turn down the opportunity and remain content(ish) with my current coif. Is it better to have loved and lost than never to have loved at all? I wondered.

Other pitfalls also loomed: What if the haircut wasn't as transformative as I dreamed? I'd be forced to accept that I already looked as good as I could. And what is the future without hope? And there was a chance that I'd embarrass myself in front of Frédéric.

All I could think of was the scene in *Educating Rita* when the heavyset, chin-hair-sprouting middle-aged woman heads to the salon gripping a picture of Lady Di and tells the stylist, "I want to look like that."

"You're really overthinking this," a friend said when I asked her—for the tenth time—if she thought I should go for it. And she was right. A few years ago (when I was truly in my late thirties), a haircut with Frédéric certainly would have been exciting, but it wouldn't have represented such a promise of rejuvenation. But now? It was as if Ponce de León himself had appeared with the E-ZPass to the Fountain of Youth.

As the big day grew closer, I felt as nervous as if I were facing risky, irreversible surgery. But at the appointed hour, wearing a carefully chosen outfit, I showed up at C.O. Bigelow ready to go under the knife. "God's Gift to Hair"—in the words of one life-style editor—had not yet arrived, so his director of education, Lisa Ferruggia, chatted me up as excitement mounted (yes, he's a hairdresser with a "director of education"). "Frédéric's like a surgeon," she told me as she arranged a tray with instruments for the great healer. Combs, brushes, glossing products. And then, just as I caught my reflection in the mirror and wished I had gotten my hair professionally blown out pre-visit, he materialized: tan, trim, and French (in a good way).

We air-kissed hello (double). "I am going to ask you a few questions," he said. He drew me close and stared at my face. "Turn left," he said, taking in my profile (the horror), "and right." Frédéric asked me to pull down my robe so he could look at my shoulders (why didn't I buy a new bra????). "What are you looking for?" he wanted to know. "Graphic? Or sexy chic, but casual." "That one," I said. "A modern shag," he responded. A hairdresser had looked into my soul. I take back everything I said earlier about stylists. Frédéric, who would probably not recognize me five minutes after the cut was done, was indeed my new B.F. He picked up his scalpel and sliced off a goiter of hair that had been growing over my right ear for years. It felt physically good, as if he'd removed a bullet. "Thank you," I said, feeling younger than I had since the Clinton administration, when Hillary was so publicly wrestling with *her* hair. Some twenty minutes later—we'd hardly had time to go through my pre-prepared small talk—Frédéric pulled out a dryer and began his tutorial. "You start with the roots," he said, "you must start with the roots." In my whole life, I'd never paid so much attention.

And then, like that, it was done. We double air-kissed again and parted ways, he to meet his public, me to start my exciting new life as an ingénue. "Your hair looks wonderful," one of C.O. Bigelow's employees told me. "Yeah," I said, feeling all thirtyish and sexy, "but I don't have much time." I could practically feel the cut growing out. She lowered her voice and passed on a tip. "Vu"—a stylist in Fekkai's New York salon—"can follow Frédéric's line, and he's only $100."

Only $100! Why, that sounded almost reasonable, if you didn't count the round-trip plane tickets from Boston, cabs to and from the airport, the hotel, and meals. I was about to come to my senses and ask what kind of woman not only pays $100 for a cut but takes an airplane to get it? Flying to another city to consult with the best heart doc—or even a plastic surgeon—is one thing, but a hairstylist? But after seeing my new do, everyone else seemed to lose their common sense, too. An acquaintance told me she had a dream about my haircut. My mother, a woman who'll drive half an hour to Costco to save a few bucks on cherry tomatoes, wanted to make an appointment. The fashion editor at the *Boston Herald* pronounced the cut "the best thing that ever happened to you," and I don't think she was kidding. "Better than meeting my husband and having my children?" I asked. "How bad did I look before?" She was silent. Moments later I was on the phone with JetBlue, looking into flights to New York. "It's like Frédéric gave you heroin," the society editor observed. "You're an addict now."

Maybe, but who can blame me? When Hillary Clinton was in her forties, she became so crazed by her hair that she thought a headband was a good idea. Years later, even after she was elected a United States senator, she was still scarred by her hair troubles as first lady. "The most important thing that I have to say today," she told Yale's class of 2001, "is that hair matters. This is a life lesson my family did not teach me, Wellesley and Yale failed to instill on me: the importance of your hair. Your hair will send very important messages to those around you. It will tell people who you are and what you stand for. What hopes and dreams you have for the world . . . and especially what hopes and dreams you have for your hair. Likewise, your shoes. But really, more your hair. So, to sum up. Pay attention to your hair. Because everyone else will."

As Melanie Griffith's character says in *Working Girl,* "you need serious hair" if you want to be taken seriously.

Well, no kidding. Researchers at Yale considered hair so crucial they studied the hair-based conclusions we draw about others. And big surprise! Women with long, straight blond hair came across as the richest and sexiest—though also self-centered and not the most intelligent. Brunettes with medium-length, casually styled hair (my namby-pamby group) were seen as good-natured and more intelligent. Women with short, highlighted hair were judged the most intelligent, confident, and outgoing. (These are obviously the ma'ams, and this is the group I'm fighting to stay out of.) I shouldn't admit this, but what I wouldn't give for long, straight blond hair—negative personality traits be darned.

Although once the blondes hit thirty or thirty-five they don't have it so easy, a friend with long blond hair complained. "I'm getting to the point where I'm wondering if I'm too old. It's making a giant statement. It could be youthful, or it could be Dolly Parton. If you start overprocessing, you can go from being a young blonde to an old blonde in one hair appointment. All it takes is for the hairdresser to bleach you out and not put in any low lights. If you don't do it right, you look cheap and old." (And you're spending a lot for the privilege. As Dolly Parton herself said, "It costs a lot of money to look this cheap.")

I know we're not supposed to set limits for ourselves, but realistically, once you've hit your mid-forties, it's probably time to accept that long blond hair—or long hair period—is never going to happen for you. Or is it? I just read that hair extensions, once only for stars, have hit the mainstream and, as the *New York Times* put it, are "an extension on youth." At prices that range from a few hundred dollars to $4,000, the plastic surgery of the hair world doesn't come cheap. And yet, with 40 percent of women over forty showing signs of female-pattern hair loss, according to the American Academy of Dermatology, the extension business is expected to thrive.

As much as $4,000 for a procedure that can actually cause hair loss and damage if not done right? It makes Frédéric himself look reasonable—and Vu a positive steal. And guess what? JetBlue was running a $25 special from Boston to New York just when I needed a cut. I convinced my best friend to meet me in Manhattan, and then convinced myself that I was just making the trip to see her, and—if I had time—I'd squeeze in a haircut with Vu. I almost would have believed it, too, had I not freaked out upon learning, the week before my appointment, that Vu had jury duty on our big day. "Sharon can cut your hair," the scheduler told me. "Everyone loves her."

Yes, I rescheduled my trip to a day when Vu would be performing his *real* civic duty—at Frédéric's Provence-inspired salon, not in some musty courthouse. Vu lived up to his billing and did indeed follow Frédéric's line, which was both good and bad, since I knew this was also a one-night stand. Even at $100, my wallet wasn't up for a long-distance relationship. As I write, more than two years have passed since my haircuts with Frédéric and Vu, and being out on my own has been rough, but I think I've Met Someone in Boston.

"So you're all set now," Ken said, relieved the searching was over. All set? Hardly. Mother Nature is not so kind. You solve one problem, and instantly another rears its aging head. As in this headline from *Marie Claire:* "Forget your hands," the magazine instructed. "These days, experts say your hair is what really betrays your age." Why? Because "we're living longer and we're torturing our hair like never before. Combine that with increased environmental insult and basic chronological aging, and you've got an epidemic of parched, brittle, and frayed 'old lady' hair."

And people thought the plague was bad.

Considering we grow new hair all the time, the concept of "aging hair" seems counterintuitive. But this "virgin" hair is not really young (just as many "virgins" aren't really virgins). Age-related scalp and follicle changes mean the hair gets less oil and melanin than it did when you were younger, and that translates to dryness, susceptibility to environmental damage, hair loss, and a bunch of other issues too disappointing to mention. I knew your hair could turn prematurely

gray. But "uneven texture" and an "increase in poros-
ity"? Those sound like challenges for the face, not the
hair. As if hair didn't already demand more than its
fair share of the grooming pie, now you've got to *eat*
with it in mind, according to New York City dermatologist Michael Lorin Reed. "If you want to keep your
hair, control your weight by exercising, not dieting,"
he told *Marie Claire*. Reed recommends consuming
high-protein, low-fat, low-carb foods. Think South
Beach diet for hair health, the magazine reported, "as
well as popping 5,000 micrograms of biotin [a B vita-
min] daily." The article concluded with advice to "use
protein-laced styling products. As your hair thins, it
gets weaker and less able to support its own weight,
leading to breakage and loss." What's next? A personal
trainer for your hair?

Just a few years ago the idea of an antiaging hair
masque was laughable, but now that the hair care
makers have taken a lesson from the skin care push-
ers and begun attaching the antiaging label to whatever
they can, there are antiaging hair vitamins and antiaging hair sunblock and antiaging hairspray. Alas, none
of these may help any more than plain old product?
As Paula Begoun, the author of *Don't Go Shopping for
Hair-Care Products Without Me*, told me, "There are
no special ingredients for 'older' hair that can improve

its texture or appearance." What it takes to make hair look good, she said, "is a combination of great hair care products [look for emollients such as cetyl alcohol in conditioners, gentle cleansing agents such as sodium lauryl sulfate in shampoos, and silicones such as cyclo-pentasiloxane in styling products, particularly those labeled "smoothing" or antifrizz]; and great styling tools [you want an implement that is easy to control and conducts heat effectively]." And, she added, "do not skimp on a great stylist." My bosom heaved as I thought of Frédéric.

But who cares if there are no special ingredients for older heads? Not consumers, apparently. Products with anti-aging vegetable proteins, antiaging sugar cane, antiaging wine extracts, you name it, are starting to show up on the shelves. What more do I need to tell you than the term "cosmeceutical" has entered the hair game? As Packaged Facts, a division of Market-Research.com, reports: "The synergies between health and appearance will drive hair care sales much more strongly in future if hair care marketers increasingly adopt and develop broader health and wellness brand positions." In spite of certain regulatory restraints, Packaged Facts says, products making promises such as "protection," "prevention," "deep cleansing," or "regeneration" are poised to fuel growth in the market segment. Or, in non-marketspeak: to sucker consumers into dropping lots of money. How much? Packaged Facts estimates that retail sales of "cosmeceutical" hair care products will approach $3.6 billion in 2010—that's up from $3 billion in 2005.

It makes me sad to think that all these fantastic antiaging claims might not be true; hair plays such a significant role in your overall antiaging game plan. Good hair, according to a new P&G Beauty study, can knock almost three years off your appearance. Three years—that's *a lot* of injectables. A senior scientist at Pantene, Lesley Bride, told me the company conducted the survey in an attempt to "understand how people view others based on how their hair looks." Uh, we choose our presidents based on hair, what more is there to say? In the survey, P&G separated women into two groups—"tidy" hair (smooth, with no tangles or dry ends) versus messy hair (frizzy and unkempt). "We took pictures of these women and then had people who didn't know them rank the photos for age and attractiveness," Bride said. On average, "tidy" hair made the models look 2.8 years younger, and upped their attractiveness scores from 4 to 6.5 (on a scale of 0–10). So one obvious take-home lesson is to brush your hair. But there's another: Bride mentioned data showing that people looked four to five years younger from the back. In other words, you may want to start entering rooms rear first. Meanwhile, since Bride spent so much time looking at hair-related data I thought I'd find out what tips she gleaned from her work. "It's made me spend more time on the back of my hair," she said. "I was like, 'I don't see the back, I don't care,' but now I know people are looking at it and making all these decisions about me."

Okay, so to summarize what we've learned: all you need is the right cut, good color, and smooth tidy hair, right? If only. Here's one last thing to keep in mind: If your hair looks too young, it could set unrealistic expectations for your face, thereby making you look older. It's almost enough to make a girl go in and get a boring, efficient haircut just to have it done with. And yet, to give up, to accept a middle-aged style, to let others pigeonhole you as "past your prime," is to do yourself a disservice. Because, as the sage Ivana Trump noted, "gorgeous hair is the best revenge."

5.

Age Is the New Fat

After 40 a woman has to choose between losing
her figure or her face. My advice is to
keep the face and stay sitting down.
—BARBARA CARTLAND

You're a toothpick." "No, I'm a moose." That's
how my friends and I used to greet each other.
Never "Hello" or "What's up?" It was always, "You're
a twig," or "Look how tiny you are." The "moose"
would deflect the compliment by extolling the slim-
ming wonders of her outfit, often black pants and a
black turtleneck. Now? For starters, none of us would
dream of wearing a black turtleneck without a splash of
color, preferably near the face. And our current saluta-
tion has little to do with BMI. It's always "Your skin

looks amazing. What are you using?" Or "You could pass for thirty-two. Really. I'm not just saying that to make you feel good."

Don't get me wrong. Being likened to a sliver of wood is still highly desirable. The problem is that slim is no longer enough; it's merely a starting point. In addition to being trim, you also have to look healthy, vibrant, and alive, darn it. The bar, always high, has been raised yet again. As no less an authority than Bobbi Brown has proclaimed: "It's not about being skinny. It's about being strong. Your clothes size and what you see in the mirror is less important than what's going on inside." You spend your whole life trying to whittle your body down, and then, when you hit forty or so, they go and change the rules on you. Now thin isn't glamorous, it's aging. "I've had to discipline myself not to run more than five miles a day," a fifty-four-year-old socialite complained, "or my face will get that horrible weathered look."

As for me, I'm almost nostalgic for the days when I was obsessed with losing weight. What an optimistic time that was, when my goal was achievable. Not *achieved*, mind you, but not a literal impossibility, either, as is my current objective—to "defy" my age. I'm fighting a moving target and an ever-growing enemy. Valerie Monroe, the beauty director of *O* magazine, captured the hopelessness of the war perfectly. "You can do something that will make you look better for a while," she told me, "but it's much more futile than anything else. Ultimately you're always going to look older every minute. Whatever you do, you have to do it again, or do something else." She paused to let it all settle in. "That's partly why I haven't done anything, because my feeling is that if I do one thing, something else is going to go and I'll have to do that. It's like standing in quicksand."

And we're all getting sucked in. I called a longtime Weight Watchers veteran, who, despite the fact that she remains "ten pounds shy of a Lane Bryant credit card," still believes thin is out there for her in this lifetime. "With weight, there's always hope. Think about what people say. 'I'm going to get skinny for my wedding.' 'I'm going to get skinny for my vacation.' 'I'm going to get skinny when I dump my boyfriend.' 'I'm going to get skinny for when I start my new job.' But you don't say, 'I'm going to get *younger* for my next vacation.' It's a completely different paradigm. I'm not skinny. I've never been skinny, but I always think I'm going to be there someday. But with age, it's not the same formula. You can't get younger. There's no 'Age Watchers.' How would it even work? When you go to a weigh-in at a Weight Watchers meeting, you take off your shoes, your belt, you don't eat right before the weigh-in, you do everything you can to get your weight down. But there's no equivalent for reducing the years. That's why we buy all that crap, and try to have an edgy haircut and youthful clothes. But still, you're forty-six years old and everyone knows it. You can't lose years."

She's right, but you could be forgiven for forgetting that inconvenient truth, considering that there's a multibillion-dollar industry trying to convince us otherwise. In fact, the term used to sell us all these products—antiaging—should tell us all we need to know about the futility of the pursuit. As the cultural critic Margaret Morganroth Gullette said when I used the words during an interview, "If you don't put 'antiaging' in quotation marks, it will subliminally argue that you believe in it. There is no such thing as 'antiaging medicine,' as many gerontologists have noted." She went on: "I doubt that the people who sell the products believe that they actually reverse the aging process. They can't, as there is no such thing. But the people who buy them may believe such a fantasy. And supporting that fantasy—even in the terms we use—that seems to me quite cruel."

Meanwhile, it's not just the plastic surgeons, cosmetics makers, and aestheticians out for our business. In this day and (anti)age, gynecologists, dentists, and even candy manufacturers have reinvented themselves as "antiaging" specialists. "Antiaging!" is the new "fat free!" or "low calorie!" Look for it on shelves near you. As Nancy Mills, a project manager with Kline & Company, a worldwide consulting and research firm, put it, advertisers use that one term—"antiaging"— and vulnerable women snap up the product. When I reached Mills she was fresh off a three-month immersion in the "internal beauty" or "nutri-cosmetics" market, and still reeling from chutzpah overload. "All of a sudden they found this new way to make any kind of product imaginable into a beauty product, so anything that is consumable can now be marketed as having beauty benefits." I asked Mills for examples of the more ludicrous products she's seen, which, knowing me, I'll be using soon enough. "Let's see, there's collagen-infused marshmallows from Japan, antiwrinkle jams from France, beauty ice cream, available only in Japan, beauty waters—" When she got to that last one she just had to interrupt herself. "Hello!" she called out sarcastically. "Water is supposed to help your skin anyway. It helps all of your organs. Why does it need to be *beauty* water?"

"Because then Borba can call it 'Age Defying Skin Balance Water' and sell it to you for $3 a bottle," I suggested. By the way, Mills was referring to the beauty water you drink, *not* the $95 beauty water you shower with. If you want that, look for the "Beauty Water Shower Purification System." Mills's litany, which included tablets that allegedly improve postmenopausal skin and others to optimize your tan, reminded me of a law named for Malcolm Muggeridge, the English journalist and social critic for the satirical British magazine *Punch*. "There is no way that a writer of fiction can compete with real life for its pure absurdity," it states. Mills had begun imagining how existing products could be repositioned to exploit aging and beauty fears. "How about curtains because they block out UV rays, or a telephone headset that doesn't clog your pores? Soon there will be beauty pillows." I had to stop her there. "Those actually exist." A few days earlier on the Web, I'd come across the Hollywood Beauty Pillow, a narrow X-shaped cushion aimed at keeping the face free from wrinkle-causing contact. "We're chasing this dream of eternal youth," Mills said. "At the last firm I worked for, they joked about 'postponing the appearance of death.' That was the little insider joke."

It would be an exaggeration to say that in the smackdown between calories and wrinkles, the antiaging concerns have triumphed. But the fact that we've now got "good fats" and "good carbs" tells you something about our priorities. As does the fact that chocolate—once *the* poster food for appearance problems—has been reborn as an antiaging elixir. "Yes, I ate the whole bar, but at 70 percent pure cacao, that's almost like eating Restylane." "Beauty-bingeing"—wolfing down formerly forbidden avocados and nuts and olive oil all in the name of blessed youth—is apparently such a concern that Hershey's provides an alcohol-company-style advisory on its website. "In case you haven't heard," it reads, "the cocoa bean contains the same natural flavanol antioxidants found in green and black teas, red wine, blueberries and more. What this means for you is that not only does dark chocolate taste great, but it might be good for you too. But keep in mind that dark chocolate is an indulgent treat, and that moderation is key when it comes to maintaining a healthy lifestyle." In other words, please gorge responsibly.

An Elizabeth Grady newspaper ad that ran in 2007 captured the weight vs. age tension perfectly: "We take the wrinkles out of weight loss," it read. "When you lose weight, you also lose skin tone. That's why those fine lines and wrinkles appear." The cure? One of Elizabeth Grady's antiaging facials, at about $115 a pop. Reflecting on the confusing times in which we live, the writer Patricia Marx, who says she has the gallbladder of a twenty-three-year-old, told me that her sense of fashion is "handicapped" because she's always been obsessed with trying to look as thin as she can, but recently a friend told her: "It's time you stopped worrying about looking fat and started worrying about looking old."

In fact, it may be time to start updating the quotes. When I came across the Duchess of Windsor Wallis Simpson's "You can't be too rich or too thin" line recently, it seemed as dated as a camera-less cell phone. Now "too thin" is bad, as the *Desperate Housewives* stars learned when they were collectively pummeled for being so skinny. "What on earth is happening to those housewives in Wisteria Lane?" the *Daily Mail* of London asked on February 23, 2006. "Marcia Cross (Bree), Teri Hatcher (Susan), Felicity Huffman (Lynette) and Eva Longoria (Gabrielle) are now bone-people with bright, tight designer clothes covering their skeletal bodies. . . . Does no one on the set mention that its stars are in danger of losing their sex appeal?"

And remember Jean Kerr's famous observation: "I'm tired of all this nonsense about beauty being only skin deep. That's deep enough. What do you want—an adorable pancreas?" That seems so quaint, doesn't it? I don't know about you, but I *do* want an adorable pancreas. And while I'm at it, a hot spleen, and a liver that turns heads. The quest for inner beauty has come so far that in 2007, Metamucil, the bulk-producing laxative and fiber supplement around since 1937, repositioned itself as a beauty product. It made its packaging pink and adopted a new slogan: "Metamucil: Beautify your inside." I'm so eager to take advantage of every "I'm getting old and losing my looks" opportunity I almost wish I had a regularity problem.

Considering that marshmallow makers are tying to get in on the antiaging game, it should come as no big shocker that health clubs are also trying to take advantage, but even so, I was surprised when I saw a *New York Times* headline asking "Who's Older, You or Your Body?" The September 26, 2006, article reported that some gyms are offering "body age" reduction plans to lure new members. The next morning I awoke with vigor I hadn't felt since high school, and I started looking for a local gym that offered either the Polar BodyAge System (developed by the heart monitor company) or the RealAge Workout (created by physician Dr. Michael Roizen). True, I already belong to a gym, and I'd have to pay a new initiation fee, but the way I look at it, if you amortize it on a per-years-dropped basis, I'd be saving money.

"I'm going to look like a teenager in a few months," I told Ken, "or at least my torso will." I was kidding, but on the way to the gym I worried that I was making trouble for myself. How could I have a mid-forties face on top of a young adult's body? I was still thinking about the looming disconnect when I arrived at the gym and was put to work filling out a questionnaire about my health and sunblock and driving and eating and drinking habits. The fitness manager weighed me, tested my cardiovascular capacity on a stationary bike, and had me sit with my legs straight out and (try to) touch my toes. He fed his results and my self-reported data, most of it true-ish, into his computer. After a few agonizing moments, it spat out its verdict on my "BodyAge": thirty-five. That was ten years younger than my so-called chronological age, but my heart sank. You know how mainstream clothing chains finally awakened to designers' vanity sizing and cleverly turned size 8 women into delighted size 4s? Well, I figured the same downsizing gimmick was at work here, which meant that thirty-five was nothing to text home about. I scanned the report to see where I'd gone wrong. Let's see: I was spending too much time in the sun, not lifting enough weights, eating too little fiber, and not stretching enough (at all, really).

But wait, what's this? Was there hope after all? Yes. "Beth," the assessment's conclusion read, "the following are factors that will improve your BodyAge." . . . If I worked on my weaknesses, it would be possible to reclaim a BodyAge of eighteen. Bring on my high school reunion! Truth be told, I know this "BodyAge" stuff is a marketing gimmick. Heck, it says so right on the website, which includes testimonials from fitness supervisors who are thrilled with the increased "personal training closing ratios" attainable once prospective members learn they can lose something more reviled than fat: years. "Within the first two months of our Polar BodyAge System purchase we increased our personal training closing ratio 30–40%," a supervisor in Missouri wrote. No word on how much younger the personal trainees became. But that's okay. It's hope in a Nautilus machine. Driving home, euphoric at the prospect of the teenage me in my future, I wanted to broadcast my news to the world. If only I had a bumper sticker: MIDDLE-AGED 18-YEAR-OLD ON BOARD!

After a few weeks of crowing about my potential, while at the same time not lifting more weights or stretching or eating Kashi, my joy receded. Not only wasn't I any younger, I was getting older. It was time to take action. No, not to do anything healthy; instituting real change is tiring. But I did have the energy to take another age test, which I hoped would provide another ego boost, which, in its way, would be youthifying. I went to a website called RealAge.com. Perhaps you've seen its ads: "Oprah has spoken—'You're going to want to take this test.'" Once again, this time in the privacy of my own home, I entered information about my family history of disease and my driving, smoking, drinking, exercise, and eating habits. I sat back and waited for my affirmation. Since I'd fudged a bit—all those years spent lying about my weight to StairMaster came in handy—I figured I'd be thirty-five at most. But this time around my "RealAge" wasn't 10 years younger than my "FakeAge," as it had been at the gym, but a mere 5.5 years.

Not to sound like an ingrate, but I could easily shave that many years myself. Who needs to fill out a long form to get the same result? The RealAge test is based on medical and scientific data, but the doctors omitted some important youth indicators in their calculations. Where were the truly diagnostic questions for assessing a person's "true" age? Such as: "Do you often feel other adults are older than you even when you're the same age?" "Are you competitive with siblings for parental love and attention?" "Does it surprise you when people take you seriously in your job?" "Are you still trying to figure out what you want to do when you grow up?"

Figuring I had nothing to lose (except years), I started following the RealAge tips that began filling my email inbox. I'm walking backward to burn more calories and increase coordination (to take a tidy nine years off my "age"). I'm telling more jokes (6 years), enlarging my social circle (3.5 years), watching wildlife videos and taking care of my emotional health to help reduce stress (16 years), and keeping in touch with distant family and friends (3.5 years). It's not easy tracking down addresses—"Dear Ninth Cousin Twice Removed

Ruth," I wrote in an email. "What did the cheetah say to the wildebeest? Heard any good gnus?"—but it's worth it.

Before I got so young that I no longer cared about aging issues, I thought I'd call Dr. Roizen (who, along with Dr. Mehmet Oz, has written several bestsellers, most recently *You: Staying Young: The Owner's Manual for Extending Your Warranty*) and find out why, exactly, inner health leads to outer beauty. He explained that the healthier you are, the more muscle tone you have, and the more tone you have, the better you look. Also this: "If you keep your arteries young, if you avoid inflammation, you will avoid that cause of wrinkles." Does a better reason to shun trans fats exist? And then there was the Fernando-Lamas-was-wrong reason. "Because you feel healthier, your attitude changes, and that necessarily gets you looking better."

"Is age the new fat?" I asked him. "Have we added a new obsession on top of an old one?" I was expecting him to say yes, since his whole thing is "RealAge," not "RealWeight." (That, by the way, is a concept I came up with to explain why the number on the scale doesn't reflect your accurate weight, but is merely a starting point from which to subtract pounds depending on time of day, month, year, clothing, recent soy sauce consumption, hair length, etc.) But Dr. Roizen instantly took issue with my use of the word "obses-sion." "The reason you're wrong and scientifically in-correct is that we are hard-wired for outer beauty," he said. "It's not a socially learned skill." Outer beauty, he explained, is an indicator of the vigor necessary to propagate the species. I asked him if he'd consider people who get Botox and face-lifts "obsessed," and he said no. "That's a genetic projection of how they look," he replied, "and that projection is giving them the con-fidence to exist." I wrote down what he said to use as ammunition against Ken. I'd position injectables as a matter of life or death.

Incidentally, during the interview Dr. Roizen's computer was acting up, and as time went on with no relief from tech support, he became increasingly and understandably frustrated, calling out to his assistant, trying his password numerous times, complaining that the machine was locking him out, until finally I asked if the stressful situation was, you know, aging. "Yes," the guru said. "It's making me older."

When I heard myself ask that question, I realized that my transformation was complete. It's official: There is no event that doesn't prompt me to think of the aging implications. This marks a switch from my former mind-set, in which all of life was viewed in weight-loss terms: You're distraught over a breakup?

Think how thin you'll get. You were up all night with food poisoning, vomiting and suffering from diarrhea? Don't brag.

Of course, there are times when one goal comes into conflict with another, a stressful dilemma faced frequently by a friend so antiwrinkle-focused that she's willing to carry an umbrella on a sunny day, thereby sacrificing her current appearance for her future looks. Last winter, for example, she had a terrible ailment. "So there I was in the throes of it," she recalled, "complete with sore throat, runny nose, the whole nine, and I shuffle to the medicine cabinet in the foolish belief that I would have medicine there. Which I didn't, because the medicine cabinet is crammed with everything but drugs. There's the vitamin E wrinkle mask; the vitamin C patches for around my eyes; Retinol cream for wrinkles; antioxidant hair mask; ginger body soak—you get the picture. I may be felled by germs, but my pores breathe free. But it's way too cold to go to CVS, and I find myself thinking, 'Well, maybe I could put the vitamin C patches in boiling water and leach out a sort of tea.' And I stopped myself—not because I thought it wouldn't work, but because I'd rather have scurvy than waste a wrinkle-fighter."

The commodity I can't stand to squander is time, which has led to some nerve-racking workout decisions of late: Burn calories? Or years? I used to come down solidly in the former category, but then I spoke to Boston posture guru Zayna Gold, who got me so scared about what a slump could do—add a tidy ten years to my look—that I was willing to forgo a day of cardio in hopes of taking a decade off my stance. Gold told me that slouching can lead to dowager's hump, potbelly, varicose veins, swayback, a double chin even. In other words, standing erect while others hunch confers an advantage even the best face-lift can't achieve, and yet no one wants to take the time to learn. We're too busy trying to look young to actually look young.

But not me. I walked into Boston Body's Newton Pilates studio uncharacteristically upright, pulling the postural equivalent of skipping breakfast before the doctor's office weigh-in. Gold, the director of the studio, is a gentle soul, but a professional who knows it's not in the client's interest to get away with a con job. "I need to see your 'global body,'" she said, circling me and issuing her verdict. "You don't have *horrible* posture." I slumped with joy! The first step to good posture is balancing properly, Gold said, which means putting your weight right behind the balls of your feet. She placed her hands on my abdomen and the small of my back and helped me suck my lower abs up and toward the back of my rib cage. "Now let out a breath while you say 'ha,'" she said. The effect was to raise and slim my torso. I was a ballerina, a veritable swan! I looked in the mirror. Not quite Margot Fonteyn, but not quite me, either. "Is it my imagination?" Gold asked, "or do you look thinner?" "Now walk," she said, letting go. I took one step and collapsed back into my old self. "Habits you've created make it impossible for you to correct your posture on your own," she explained. "You don't feel where you're going wrong." Short of traveling with Gold attached, what can be done? She prescribed core-strengthening exercises. True, those sound tiring and time-consuming, but there's good news: "One way to strengthen core muscles in order to stand better is to stand better." As you would imagine, Gold has wonderful posture, but even she has issues. "I'll be sitting at a holiday meal and it looks as if I'm trying to pose. I wish I could slump."

Perhaps that's where my destiny lies—at the forefront of a backlash. Think of it: Perfect posture looks too posed, Botoxed faces appear emotionless, plastic surgery can pull too tight—but we Backlashers are the real deal. Perhaps I can whip together a protest, picketing the Oscars' red carpet, carrying signs in support of natural aging. Years from now, grateful women will commemorate our watershed moment, the Slouch on Hollywood.

6.

The Absolute(ish) Truth

One should never trust a woman who tells
her real age. If she tells that,
she'll tell anything.
—OSCAR WILDE

You know what I can't stand? When a comment sounds admiring, but upon analysis proves to be an affront. (This is a productive way to spend your time, picking apart everything that's said to you.)

Here's the kind of "accolade" I mean: "Wow! You look amazing."

My education in why this was an insult struck not long after I'd been hired by the local Fox TV affiliate. Every week I'd go on the 5 P.M. newscast and banter with the anchor about the important things: the awkwardness of the triple air kiss, people who use sunglasses as a crutch, bra-induced back-fat bulges. You get the idea. *The NewsHour with Jim Lehrer* it wasn't, but playing a TV commentator on TV was fun, and my two-minute gig would have been the ideal freelance job had it not been for the small matter of finances. Because there was absolutely no way I would appear on television looking anything like the actual me, I was forced (by me) to hire hair and makeup professionals before every newscast. Whenever I'd admit this extravagance to people, they were surprised. "The station doesn't have someone who does that?" they'd ask. No. In my experience, on most local shows you're on your own. Although I could never bring myself to do the math, I knew that my grooming costs were outpacing my earnings. I was spending something on the order of $25 a minute to *work*. And that wasn't even counting the tip for the shampoo girl or the growing problem of "glamour creep."

What's glamour creep? This: Once I saw how much prettier, sexier, and younger I looked with a blow-out and expertly applied eye base, it became hard for me to go to any "event"—a preschool soccer game—undone. That sounds vain, I know, but it might have happened to you, too, if you'd become a walking before-and-after demonstration the way I had. The disparity was so pronounced that even a five-year-old could tell the difference. "Sonia didn't believe that was *you* on TV!" Sonia's mother reported one day, a bit too cheerfully. Her daughter, she said, could not recognize me as the same person she saw daily dropping off my son at kindergarten.

But Sonia was the least of my problems. One day I was sitting around the Fox studio with the crew waiting for my live shot when the producer, a twenty-seven-year-old cutie with young hair and no collagen issues, asks the cameraman his age. Turns out he's thirty-five. "I thought you were in your twenties," I said. He was thrilled, but what a tactical error on my part. Even a rookie trial lawyer knows you don't introduce a subject into testimony unless your client can withstand cross-examination. As they say in the courtroom, I'd "opened the door."

Grabbing her opportunity, the producer pounced: "How old are *you*, Beth?" My alarm must have shot heat waves across the room. Because she'd only seen "TV Me," I was pretty sure she thought I was younger than I am, and I was sad that my cover was about to be blown. "I'm sorry," she said quickly, "you don't have to tell me."

Of course I didn't, and yet, in 2007, playing coy isn't cool. Where had I gone so wrong? I was turning into—had *turned* into—precisely the kind of "girl" I'd pitied as a child. I'd see them by the pool on trips to Miami Beach, leather-skinned, liver-spotted, sun reflectors positioned just so, as they coyly claimed to be "39" or "39a." And here I was, thirty-five years later, better informed about UV rays, but in the end, no more evolved in the self-acceptance realm.

But what age should I claim to the producer? The seconds ticked by as I pondered a number to throw out. This was one of the first times since I'd turned forty that I'd been asked flat out, to my face. Less out of honesty than a lack of forethought and strategy, I confessed.

That's when she launched her Scud: "Wow!" she said. "You look amazing. I thought you were in your thirties."

I should have been mentally rehearsing for my imminent banter with the anchor, but age-related neurosis consumed me. Let's see. She considered me "amazing" for being in my forties, but what was her opinion of my looks when she had me pegged for thirty-five? That I'd let myself go? I couldn't decide which was worse: to be thought dowdy but under forty, or to be admired as well preserved yet be practically old enough to be her mother. (If I'd had kids young, that is, instead of waiting until I was in my very late thirties to start, which has had the unhappy side effect of throwing me into playdate situations with women a decade or more my junior. It's not the lower back that bothers older mothers; it's the crow's-feet.)

I was swirling into my own private age-shame spiral when the news director's voice in my earpiece startled me. "Thirty seconds, Beth."

With that, the in-studio chitchat ended, and the producer never mentioned the matter again. Even so, the dreaded subject was not dead, merely dormant as it gathered strength for a second attack a few months later—*on air.* The topic of the day was a new high-pitched cell phone ring audible only to teenagers and young people. The anchor and I were riffing on a phenomenon called "aging ear"—is there no part of the body that won't turn on you?—when she said, "I'm forty-one, how old are you Beth?"

Like Gloria Steinem and Shirley MacLaine, this was a woman who embraced her age. If only more of us were like her, I thought, maybe we'd be judged for who we are—doctors, soldiers, mothers, volunteers—rather than by our wrinkles. I was building up a good head of feminism when I realized that rather than applaud the anchor's self-assurance, as I'd been pretending to myself, I resented it. Women like her make women like me feel even worse. I had no choice but to answer the question. To demur in the face of her emotion-free statement of fact would be worse than any number could be, no matter how high. "I'm forty-four," I said, hoping I sounded like it didn't bother me at all, as simple a statement of fact as my name.

The anchor played the cell phone ring for viewers and then asked me what—if anything—I'd heard. "My mother's voice telling me I shouldn't have said my age on TV."

Everyone cracked up, but as I was walking home, the incident started to bother me. As a print journalist—and, more important, a formerly young person who carelessly let time pass, and now look at the predicament I'm in—I'd never worried about workplace age discrimination, and yet one of the reasons I wanted to keep my fortysomethingness quiet was that TV is generally a young woman's game. I was afraid that once the truth was out I could no longer be considered current or hip, no matter what I said. But it wasn't only the age-discrimination angle that was bothering me. Once the specter of lying had been raised, there were practical matters to consider: How many years should I shave?

I pulled out my middle-aged cell phone, with its basic ringtone and unused text-message function, and called a friend who was toying with the idea of lying to her own children about her age. It wasn't them she was trying to impress, but the other mothers in the preschool. She hoped her kids would pass along her "age" to their little friends and it would filter up to the moms, all of whom were much younger than she. Even as my friend looked forward to her new (fictional) younger self, she fretted about creating a trust issue that would last a lifetime. "And for what?" she asked. "I'm not going to pretend to be *significantly* younger. I'm going through all this mental anguish and dishonesty for a two-year boost."

On the one hand she was right: a measly two years. Not enough to make a difference to anyone but her. And yet, while I didn't want to encourage her, I knew the deception might be worth it. Properly executed, a two-year exfoliation can be turned into a ten-year savings. I learned that strategy from a particularly cunning friend when she was forty-one. Well, she was forty-three, but out of respect I'll report her stated age, since those particular two years perfectly illustrate the genius of her ploy. "If you are forty-three," she explained, "you're only two years away from forty-five, which is horrifying because it's that much closer to fifty. So by shaving off a mere two years, you're really getting about ten, because at forty-one, you're just skimming forty."

Think of it as Math for Women of a Certain Age.

The idea is to cling to the previous decade as long as possible, remaining in your "late thirties" well into your mid-forties, at which point you switch to "forty-ish" and hang on to that as long as you can, then around your fiftieth birthday admit to fortysomething, and repeat throughout the decades. If anyone challenges you, you can point to a *New Yorker* cartoon from 2005 that shows a man and a woman sitting at a bar having a drink. "They say the early forties is the new late thirties," he tells her.

Or you may want to use a variation of the Bob Hope line: "She said she was approaching forty and I couldn't help wondering from what direction."

I met my mathematician friend for coffee recently and noticed her finger was in a splint. She'd broken it "skiing," she said. "I'm sorry," I said. "When did it happen?" Long pause. "Four weeks ago, but I'm telling everyone last weekend, so it doesn't seem like I'm taking forever to heal, like an old person does." And technically she didn't fall skiing, but when she tripped walking. "What you want to create," she coached, "is a picture of perfect youthful vitality."

She spelled out her technique, and it sounded as if she were teaching a class for covert agents. "Your goal is to create a whole new identity," she instructed. You want to be thought of as a person who knows Paul

McCartney from his Starbucks years, not as one of the founding members of the Beatles; someone who's familiar with the Brady Bunch from the movie, not the original run of the prime-time series. "Don't talk about anything you really want to talk about. Hot flashes, how long it takes to stretch out in the morning, which procedures you want. Keep your mouth shut. You talk about what young people talk about. The gym, concerts, food—but not with any sort of mind toward health. You can discuss anything but what's on your mind, like 'How do I make these brown spots go away.' Once they know your age," she warned, "any opinion you have or observation you make will be filtered through the lens of 'This person is old and doesn't know what's going on.'"

But maintaining a false identity can be tricky. She recently blew her cover, she said, while making conversation with an intern who'd moved into a new apartment. "Did you get your new phone number yet?" my friend asked. "What do you mean 'new phone number'?" the intern said. "I'm using my cell."

As my pal spoke, I recalled advice I'd gotten from a sixty-year-old clothing model a number of years ago. On shoots she spends a lot of time with younger people, and in an attempt to fit in, she's disciplined herself to never make a reference that's more than two years old, or refer to anything she's done in the past. "Kids don't want to hear about the 'old days,'" she said, putting quotation marks around the verboten term.

There's no rest for the weary, is there? I've read about thirty-three-year-olds throwing themselves high-profile *thirtieth*-birthday bashes, classmates banding together to collectively forward-date the year of their graduation, an unmarried menopausal socialite who kept tampons in her medicine cabinet to fool suitors into thinking she was still fertile. One woman, a contemporary when we met in 1983, engages in relentless age management, clipping the years as one would a lawn, so as to keep it a constant.

"I lie so often about my age that I actually have to do the math with my birth date to figure out how old I really am," she confided recently. "I've decided to stay at 38—believable, I feel (you go too young and it's a stretch), and by now, the number just flies off my lips. 'Why, yes, I'll admit to 38,' I say. I find that if you do this for several years straight, you slip off the track of Real Age and into the groove of whatever number you pick. Former peers (now 45) complain about perimenopause symptoms and thinning hair, and I reply soothingly, 'Oh, I hope I look that good when I'm your age.'

"And while I constantly lie, I keep my 'landmark' people at their real ages. For instance, my brother is 52, chronologically 7 years older. But since I'm 38 now, he's 14 years older. People comment on the great gap in our births. I'd rather have the label of 'accident' than 'fortysomething.'"

(She subscribes to the George Costanza school of subterfuge. "It's not a lie if you believe it.")

I was nodding along, awed by her diligence, when I realized there are Six Ages of Woman: the age she wants to be; the age she claims to be; the age she thinks she looks; the age *others* think she looks; the age kindly friends tell her she looks; and, oh yes, her chronological age. Ideally you want to keep the numbers within striking—or lying—distance.

But here's a question to ponder: If you *look* a particular age, what difference does the number you report to others mean? A lot, maybe. Research done by marketing experts on "price endings" suggests that people react so emotionally to numbers that $19.99 feels much less expensive than $20. Studies have repeatedly found a greater perceived difference in cost between items priced at $19.99 and $24.99 than those priced at $20 and $25, even though it's $5 in each case. There's something about that initial "1" that tricks people. "We know it has to do with the left-most digit," Robert Schindler, professor of marketing at Rutgers University at Camden, told me.

"Why does this happen?" he asked rhetorically. "We're in the realm of speculation, but it's interesting. It looks like there are two parts of our mind. The part that's intellectual knows that $19.99 and $24.99 are five dollars apart, just as $20 and $25 are. But there is another part of our mind, that we might call emotional, that also puts thoughts into our heads. The current philosophers are calling it 'system one' and 'system two' processes. The more primitive is system one. It roughly corresponds to heart vs. mind, but that simplifies it too much. System one is more than just emotions, it's thought and feeling, although that thought is not very organized. It's more like the thought of a primitive mammal, so it makes mistakes. It overweights the leftmost digit. Some of us know what's going on, yet the effect happens anyway."

The lesson: In a society gone self-branding mad, in which we are "the CEOs of our own companies: Me Inc."—to quote business management guru Tom Peters—perhaps only a fool doesn't "price" herself advantageously. My new age: 39.99.

So that's the lesson from business types. What does a psychologist who's an antiaging expert suggest? Basically the same thing. "If you're between thirty and eighty you should lie," Michael Brickey, the president of the Ageless Lifestyles Institute and author of

Defying Aging and *52 Baby Steps to Grow Young,* told me. Why? Because "when you tell someone your chronological age, they pull out their stereotypes of that age, and those are usually based on how their parents' generation acted at that age. And this generation is aging much better, looking younger, and living longer."

And, frankly, the young have no idea what they're talking about, specifically when it comes to when middle age, or even old age, starts. A study published a number of years ago in the *Journal of Gerontology* proves the point (and also makes a secondary point, which is that men are faster to brand women "middle-aged" than women are): male college students set the onset of middle age for a woman at 35.6; female college students said it begins 37.9. Meanwhile, the older study subjects reported that middle age doesn't start for a woman until she's 40.3 (according to men) and 43.5 (according to women). That's not great, but since the British euphemism "middle youth"—to describe the 35-to-45-year-old crowd—has not caught on here, we'll take what we can get.

My thought is that Dr. Brickey is right—best to keep your number to yourself. If that proves impossible, he recommends this tactic: "Think of yourself as many ages—with your repertoire of ages becoming richer every year. For example, there are times when you want to get down on the floor and play with kids like you are a kid yourself, times when you want to play ball like a twenty-year-old, and times when you want to give mature sagely advice. Being many ages lets you choose the age that fits the occasion. When people ask your age, you often feel like they are filling out a checklist. Tell them you are many ages and you get an interesting conversation."

Or they'll flee.

Either way you win. One of my favorite pieces of advice comes from one of the loveliest women I've met recently, Cornelia Guest, the daughter of the late socialite and gardener C. Z. Guest. Cornelia was "debutante of the decade" back in the 1980s, so her age is sort of guessable—actually, you could look it up—but even so, she insists on never "attaching a number" to herself. "Society looks so harshly at people now," Guest told me. "We're so quick to throw people away. After people get to a certain number [nobody] cares about them anymore."

I thought about all the magazine cover stories I'd seen promising "Good skin at any age! What to do when you're in your twenties, thirties, forties, and fifties." This so-called any age ends at fifty-nine. After that, you're on your own. Good luck!

"There's such paranoia about age now," Lynne Luciano Loeb, the social historian, told me. "People are so frightened of it. Apparently it has very little to do with the fear of death—it strikes at age thirty. At thirty, people are not looking into the abyss of their mortality." No, but they are looking into the abyss of laugh lines. And in this day and age, that's pretty scary, too.

Americans are living longer than we ever have—life expectancy for a child born in the U.S. has gone from 69.6 in 1955 to 77.9 for a child born in 2005—but the age at which we're made to feel old is getting younger. Even for supermodels. Here's what supermodel Gisele Bündchen told the *London Sun* a few years ago, when she was all of twenty-five years old: "I definitely feel that I had more men hitting on me in the past. When I was younger, maybe 15 or 16, for sure. Maybe I am not as good looking. I don't know."

It's now five years later and my guess is that as thirty looms, twenty-five is starting to look pretty good. And it's always the way. Remember my friend the "forty-one"-year-old who was trying to stay as far from fifty as possible? She's "fifty-one" now (fifty-three, really) and trying to avoid any association with the number sixty, which in a few short years will look terrific as she heads toward seventy.

And so on.

Meanwhile, as the lying continues, we need to ask ourselves a question: Whom, exactly, are we trying to impress? Friends and family are out—they already know your real age. Deceiving acquaintances is tempting but risky. If you let your guard down and become pals, how do you explain your high school friends are all much older than you? Ditto if you meet a guy through an Internet dating service who's *somehow* under the impression you're ten years younger than you are. Sometimes lying to random young strangers holds allure, but considering that most kids don't really notice anyone above twenty-five years old, why bother? And yet, a fortysomething I know, who shall remain nameless (if, alas, not ageless), is constantly on the prowl for "youth validation." She's endlessly angling to be carded by the clerk at the liquor store, complimented on her skin tone by the aesthetician, considered a peer by her teenage daughter's friends. "No one ever gives me what I'm looking for," she says. She wishes she didn't care so much, but she does. "It's as if being young is an accomplishment," she told me. "And if you're not young, it's because you've done something wrong. When I tell people my age, I feel like I'm admitting to a personal weakness."

So in the end, what do you do if someone asks you flat out for your age? Mary Schmich, the *Chicago Tribune* columnist and Brenda Starr author, has a good comeback: "Like many women my age, I am twenty-eight years old." But I also like this response from the author of *The Metrosexual Guide to Style: A Handbook for the Modern Man.* "I've stopped answering that question with a numerical answer," Michael Flocker emailed me. "I find it's much more comforting to say I'm the same age as Brad Pitt and Johnny Depp."

As for me, on my next birthday, I'll be turning Meg Ryan.

7.

How to Look "Natural" in Three Hours or Less

In the factory we make cosmetics,
in the drugstore we sell hope.
—CHARLES REVSON

Some women are yo-yo dieters. Me, I'm a yo-yo makeup wearer. So wild are my grooming swings that on many days, unless Chapstick counts, I leave the house cosmetics-free, and on others I'm late getting my kids to school because I'm priming my lashes. In a delinquent period I'll think nothing of appearing at luncheons, cocktail parties, interviews, without so much as tinted moisturizer. But then something will jolt me out of my slovenliness. Maybe a professional makeup artist will do my face for TV and I'll notice that, wow, I can still look perky. Or I'll read a study showing that women who wear makeup are more likable than their un-"done" counterparts. Or I'll catch sight of my pallor in a store mirror. Then, as quickly as a Bloomingdale's cosmetics saleswoman can ask "What are you doing for lip this fall?" a mania will set in, and I'll buy products that seem almost intended to mock the purchaser: a reverse eyeliner for $24; a colorless priming pencil; a $35 "eyebrow enhancer" that conditions the aging and thinning brow; a tub of "instant-action" antifatigue beauty booster. As far as I could see, the only thing that happened instantly when I fell for that last one was an $85 charge appearing on my Visa bill.

I'm pretty sure none of the invisible glamour enhancers or flesh-colored lip pencils or nude eye shadows I've bought has improved my appearance in any way. But the problem is that I can't be totally, 100 percent positive they didn't. I spend good money on these items for the same reason disbelievers pass along chain letters: as protection against the big What If. My friends use these pointless products—What If they're gaining an antiaging advantage? Besides, I'm an optimist at heart, and when it comes to cosmetics, I follow Samuel Johnson's observation about second marriages: a triumph of hope over experience. I'm convinced a skin-tightening, dark-circle-banishing wonder product is poised to hit the market. In fact, no sooner do I come to terms with the failure of a foundation, lip liner, or instant eye-lift pencil (I won't ask how something you *draw* with can lift your eyes) than I get wind of one that's new and improved. Often I'll get the pitch from the same cosmetics lady who sold me the product I'd just discarded. "*This* one is amazing," she'll say. Soon enough I'll find myself succumbing to the four phases of the department store makeover: (1) Wow! (2) Buy everything they've got. (3) Go home to duplicate what the makeup artist did. (4) Huh?

My goal in this hyperluminescent age is for my face to give off as much light as a baseball stadium during a night game. If I'm properly made up, looking directly at me should be as retina-frying as staring into the sun during an eclipse. But that, of course, remains elusive. Between the mascara, eyeliner, concealer, blush, and illuminating cream, my face ends up a pearlescent smudged mess. Lacking the one product I do know how to use—makeup remover—I end up going through a roll of toilet paper trying to get it all off. My new, downsized goal: simply to have my own clean face back.

After falling for the flattery job approximately one zillion times, I asked cosmetics cop Paula Begoun, the author of *Don't Go to the Cosmetics Counter Without Me,* how to tell when you're being duped. "As a general rule," she emailed, "it is safe to assume you are always being conned." Despite thousands of *topical* products that claim to work miracles, she noted, plastic surgeons and cosmetic dermatologists are not going out of business. "It doesn't take much for a woman to be convinced to buy a skin care product or makeup item," she continued. "We want to believe the hype, no matter how many times we are disappointed. Cosmetics salespeople are trained to sound convincing about their products, but more often than not they have no idea what they are talking about." They bandy about terms like "antioxidants," "free radical damage," or talk about results of research, and "when pressed for details or facts they simply make less and less sense. But it really doesn't matter what they say, women tend to believe them."

I was in one of my cosmetic-depressive phases (my default position) when the press release arrived announcing Bobbi Brown's "Looking your best at 50 and beyond" session at the upcoming AARP convention. By the way, I wrote "AARP" and not "American Association of Retired Persons" because the organization formally changed its name to initials only in 1999 since half its members actually work. The antiaging craze has become so pervasive that (a) no one can retire anymore; and (b) even a group that represents people in the back half of life feels the need to distance itself from the repulsive act of getting older. Like KFC (né Kentucky *Fried* Chicken) before it, the AARP wants to keep prospective consumers' minds off a certain unspeakable word.

Bobbi Brown's talk started at 12:30. I figured I'd hit the Hello! Skinny Jeans convention booth and then saunter into the cosmetics session around 12:25 and grab a seat. Except that when I arrived, a mob was trying to push its way into the room, which already appeared to be way above the stated 586-person capacity. Those who'd come too late to get seats were happily standing. Lower-back problems, bunions, arthritis, varicose veins, none of it mattered. When you're about to learn four simple steps to a nonsurgical face-lift from a cosmetics icon, physical discomfort is secondary. I was standing toward the back when Bobbi entered with her People, a small bevy of thin, stylish, young *Devil Wears Prada* New Yorkers. Later, when the Beautiful Ones went into the audience to hold cordless mikes so the AARPers could ask Bobbi their makeup questions, the distinction between what could be (the lovelies) and what was (us) was almost too painful to contemplate.

Bobbi took the stage and a few minutes into her talk issued what I've come to recognize as the standard makeup artist/style guru disclaimer: "When a woman is confident," she said, "to me, *that's* beautiful." Confidence—everyone in the beauty world pays homage. Sometimes instead of saying "confidence," they talk about "owning your look" or "knowing and liking yourself." After you hear this kind of thing often enough, you become numb to the inherent contradiction: if all it takes to make me feel good is, well, *me*, why do I need what *you're* pushing? And maybe we wouldn't be so insecure if the cosmetics companies didn't spend millions in advertising geared toward making us believe we need their products. If only Congress would hold hearings aimed at finding documents showing Big Blush intentionally addicts women to its products. They put something in the lipstick, I'm sure of it. But the beauty executives stick to the "inner confidence" line so relentlessly, and Bobbi Brown herself seemed so nice and so reasonable about the whole issue, that you come to believe that the makeup truly unlocks the latent confidence buried beneath your ghastly uneven skin tone; it's lying there, like a Monet hidden under a painting of dogs playing poker.

Bobbi has gotten her famous "Makeup Face-Lift" down to four steps. The crowd was rapt as she spelled out the routine. Number One: Use concealer to lighten your under-eye area so you look less tired. Number Two: Use a good foundation to smooth out your face. Number Three: Define your lips, eyes, and brows. These fade as you age. Number Four: Use blush to make your cheeks "pop." "A little pink looks gorgeous," she said as the audience smiled. Yes, we had jowls and deep nasolabial folds and schleppy outfits and bad hair and horrible tote bags, but with a little pink blush, we'd be magnificent.

The audience could have listened forever, but Bobbi wanted to take questions. A woman stood up and announced, by way of asking for lipstick advice, that she was seventy-five years old. The crowd went wild. I'm not sure why. Maybe they were psyched that she still cared about her appearance, or maybe they cheered because here was someone older than them. Bobbi started recommending flattering colors, but all I could think about was a smokers' rights meeting I covered a few decades ago, in a smoky VFW hall, in which a woman rose from the crowd, said she was ninety years "young," and the other smokers started cheering, as if her existence was proof that all this concern about secondhand smoke and cancer was utter nonsense. I was still thinking back to that smokers' meeting when I was jolted back to the present day by a frightening pronouncement from Bobbi.

The biggest mistake a woman can make, she warned, is wearing no makeup. The women who wear too much, she added, are much easier to help than those who do nothing. She couldn't be looking right at me, could she? A few minutes later the session was over and a small crowd gathered around Bobbi. I asked why the nonwearers were lost causes. "Very few people need nothing as we get older, and if you're wearing nothing," she said, it indicates there may be something going on in "other areas of your life." Bobbi said that over the years she's observed "a strong connection between the time a woman spends on herself and her self-esteem. Sometimes a woman doesn't wear makeup because she's juggling many different things in her life, and she puts herself and her appearance last on the list. The truth is that when you spend a little extra time on yourself, it can make you feel so much better." So the eyes aren't the window to the soul—the eyeliner is?

I wanted to protest and tell her, "I don't have psychological problems, I'm just lazy." I would have liked to point her to a study, done by psychologists at Old Dominion University, that found that the more makeup a woman wears, the worse she feels without it, and conversely, those who typically wear little makeup don't perceive a great drop in attractiveness when they're barefaced. But other women were waiting for Bobbi's attention, and the bevy of beauties kind of intimidated me, so I slunk off.

As I departed I heard the next person in line spilling her guts to Bobbi: "I'm on a never-ending quest for the right concealer," she said. "It's like my life's work."

And yet, even Bobbi knows that her four simple steps can't solve all of life's problems. Sometimes even she has to go beyond concealer and her beloved gold shimmer brick and wear a hot pink scarf as a diversion "so no one notices how fat my butt is." The crowd laughed in sympathy. "As we get older the body plumps but the face un-plumps," she added.

Bobbi's diversion comment made me realize that the professional from whom I should seek advice was not a makeup artist, but a magician. When I got the manager of Manhattan's well-known Fantasma Magic store on the line and made him understand why, exactly, I was seeking a magician's help, he offered that "misdirection is a big key in magic." And the good news, Magick Balay told me, is that it's so easy to divert someone's attention, you can actually steal a person's watch (as part of a trick) and he won't realize it's happened. How? Get people laughing, Balay advised. When the chuckler closes his eyes for a moment, Balay strikes. "Whenever I make a joke it's because I'm hiding something," he said. Take-home message: Laughter's not only the best medicine, but an effective antiwrinkle cream, too.

Later that evening, with Bobbi's diagnosis of the deeper troubles revealed by a lack of surface artifice weighing on me, I stopped into the Bobbi Brown counter at Neiman Marcus. I was on my way to a party celebrating the launch of the *Boston Globe*'s new fashion magazine, and as the "Fashion Outsider" columnist, I certainly wanted to look like I wasn't having trouble in other areas of my life. As it happened, a special makeup event was under way, which meant that one of Bobbi's national artists was on hand. The woman doing my face called her over to consult on a blush color. I was tempted to say "a little pink is gorgeous," the way Bobbi herself would have, but I kept my mouth shut. "What are you wearing tonight?" the national artist asked. "Uh, what I have on now," I said, apologetically gesturing to my basic black shirt and practical skirt. It was not, I knew, the statement of a woman who owned her look. But she smiled anyway, because if there's one thing successful makeup artists are good at, it's making each woman feel beautiful. I know because it's happened to me countless times, and I've seen other women blossom, albeit temporarily, under the praise. In the chair next to me that evening was a woman who, at first glance, appeared to be an average fifty-five-year-old woman with dull skin. I wouldn't have looked twice at her, except that the makeup artists were going on and on about her beautiful eyes and wonderful cheekbones, and the next thing I noticed, she was glowing like a thirty-five-year-old, although I couldn't tell if it was from the gold shimmer or the compliments.

Actually, it was probably both. Like hairdressers, makeup artists often double as therapists. Cece Hekman, an Armani artist working at Saks Fifth Avenue in Manhattan, told me that many women come as much for the pampering as for the cosmetics. "Having someone pay attention to them makes them feel like 'I still matter,'" she said. "The makeup works at a deeper level." She told me about customers who feel so bad about themselves they can barely stand to look in the mirror, and the others who've lost their jobs and come for the ego boost. "I always feel like I'm going to cry at work." I asked her what look everyone is trying to achieve. "To look younger," she said. "That's all they want."

What Hekman sees at her makeup counter, Judith Wright, an expert in "soft addictions," sees in the women who come to her for life coaching. "We all have these deeper hungers and needs," she said. "To matter, to be seen, to be respected, to belong, to connect, to love and be loved. But oddly, in our society we don't talk about those things. We talk about our surface wants. I want to look good, but all these deeper hungers are what's driving it. If I just wear the right makeup, then I'll be attractive and then I'll be loved." What? That's not true?

"It becomes even a bigger issue later on if a woman has always based her worth on her appearance. If she was always known as cute or hot or sexy, then that becomes her identification. You put aging in there— she gets crow's-feet or other lines, and that is very threatening to her identity. It's not just that she's losing her looks, but herself. Then you see that scramble, for makeup, cosmetic surgery, getting obsessed with her workout, wearing shorter skirts. It looks like she's trying to keep her looks, but to her, her looks and her self are one and the same."

Considering that the definition of insanity is repeating the same behavior and hoping for a different result, and taking into account that I've been getting makeup tips for twenty years and not one has taken, I thought it might be time to seek out "don'ts." *Not* doing something is something I can do. And who better to guide me than a Hollywood makeup artist skilled at making actresses look older for their roles? I'd find out what he does and steer clear. I got Tim Quinn, Armani's Celebrity Face Designer, on the phone, and within minutes he revealed a "don't" so frightening I should have put him on hold and broadcast a nationwide alert. Code Old. "The biggest mistake women make is with foundation color," he began, explaining that some women go too light, which is precisely what makeup artists do to *age* someone on screen. "We make them look pasty," he said. "As you get older you start to lose color in your face." I silently vowed to buy the darkest foundation available, but seconds later I learned that, too, was a no-no. "It's about finding a happy medium," Quinn told me. "You see people who go too tan. It makes the skin look flat. They take bronzing powder and it makes your skin look dull. It ages you. Most women are trying to get their skin as luminous as possible, then you combat that by putting flat matte bronzer all over your face." The unfairness of it all almost undid me. Here we are, trying our hardest and yet achieving the polar opposite of our goal.

Trying to keep my wits about me so I could take notes, I asked Quinn how, precisely, you know which shade is right. The aim, he explained, is continuity in color from your décolletage to your face. Go to a department store wearing an open-collar shirt, apply three stripes of different shades along your cheek and jawbone, grab a mirror, and head for natural light. "Choose the color that becomes transparent," he said. Or else!

Oh, and beware blush. Yes, a little pink looks gorgeous, but *only* if applied correctly. Wear it beneath the cheekbone if you're over thirty or so, Quinn warned, "and you can end up looking hollow. It's something we do to age somebody." And just one more little thing: Don't use too much makeup. Lipstick, lip liner, too-dark nail polish, even, can accentuate wrinkles. Got all that?

The don'ts were beginning to frighten me, so I asked for some do's. Quinn mentioned that he sometimes uses surgical tape on the back of the neck for a nonsurgical neck lift. "A lot of the old Hollywood girls do it," he told me, the "old Hollywood girls" being women in their fifties and beyond. "It's awesome. It pulls your neck taut, and it stays put. I've done it for the red carpet." It sounded so good I almost wished I had neck issues. Something to look forward to, I guess.

"And everyone I know uses false lashes," he added. "As you get older you start to lose lashes. False lashes instantly make you look younger."

False lashes. Aha! That's it—that's all that's standing between me and my rightful youthful self. I went online in search of information, but the stories I read scared me lash-less. If not done right, you can lose lashes, or the glue could burn your eyes. One woman I interviewed told me she almost glued her eyelids together with a kit bought at a discount department store. "It's a good thing I didn't apply them while driving like I do most of my makeup," she said. "That would have been hard to explain on the accident report." She never did end up wearing them. "Even though the glue was all over the lash line, I couldn't get the fake lashes anywhere near there, so instead they were stuck all crooked in the middle of the lid like a second very black, very dense, very fake layer. Sharks have extra teeth, I had extra lashes."

I decided I'd stick with, or, I should say, start using, one of the gross of mascara tubes I'd accumulated. But mascara can do a number on you, too. That's what Bobbie Weiner, a Hollywood special effects artist who worked on *Titanic*, told me. I figured a woman who turned hundreds of actors into corpses would know a thing or two about aging. As the day goes along, she said, mascara flakes can collect under your eyes and cause the dreaded darkening effect. "One of the secrets is to take a Q-tip, get some cream that doesn't burn your eyes, and wipe under the eye to get rid of the dark. That will brighten your face.

"People don't realize you shouldn't use any eye shadows that are dark once you pass that thirty-eight, forty mark," she added. "The blues, the purples, the browns. You've got to lighten everything up."

I was beginning to feel old and tired just listening, so I asked if she had any instant youth-lifts. Yes! Put your hair in a ponytail (if it's not too short), apply a bit of blush, don sunglasses, and—here's the key part—toss on that universal symbol of sportiness and youth: the baseball cap. And voilà! Or, better yet, pull an Anna Wintour, and conceal as much of your face as possible. That's 83 percent, to be precise, according to an irreverent French television show that diagrammed the *Vogue* editor's facial features and determined that she is 63 percent hair, 20 percent sunglasses, and 17 percent face. I'm sure you've seen her in shots at Fashion Week in New York. Big bangs, big glasses. Let's just hope the John Lennon look doesn't come back.

Weiner made makeup application sound so easy—just as Bobbi Brown and the others had—that I began to wonder why I go through long stretches of walking around barefaced. "I think it's because you insist on taking an all-or-nothing approach," a friend said. She suggested baby steps: tinted moisturizer, lip gloss, a tiny bit of blush. "The things that are easy to apply." I was so motivated by this new concept of moderation that I dug up a Coco Chanel quote I came across a few years ago that—briefly—made an impact on me. "I don't understand how a woman can leave the house without fixing herself up a little, if only out of politeness," she said. "And then, you never know, maybe that's the day she has a date with destiny. And it's best to be as pretty as possible for destiny."

8.

Facial Fitness:
No Pain, No Vain

The problem with beauty is that it's like being
born rich and getting poor.
—JOAN COLLINS

When skin care's the subject, former Defense Secretary Donald Rumsfeld doesn't usually spring
to mind. Secretary of State Condi Rice maybe, but not
him. And yet, if you think about it, Rumsfeld's famous
riff on "unknown unknowns" could double as ad copy
for Neutrogena. "As we know," he told the press corps
in 2002, "there are known knowns. There are things
we know we know. We also know there are known
unknowns. That is to say, we know there are some-
things we do not know. But there are also unknown
unknowns, the ones we don't know we don't know."

As in: Okay, I knew I had to worry about the wrinkles I could see, and I suspected I had to do something about sun damage lurking below the surface. But who ever thought to stress about flabby facial muscles? And yet, the threat of a ninety-eight-pound weakling of a forehead is out there—the dreaded unknown unknown.

The cosmetic "to do" list lengthens.

Your butt, it turns out, doesn't have the only cheeks that need to feel the burn to stay perky. The neck and face have approximately fifty-five muscles, and if you don't exercise them, they atrophy. That's what one of the country's top facial-fitness coaches told me. Yes, I said facial-fitness coach. To compete in today's world, your forehead needs a personal trainer.

I wish I'd let this regimen stay one of those unknown unknowables. Because even though I'm not satisfied with my current skin care routine, at least the only energy required is unscrewing a jar lid or forking over my credit card.

But facial exercise showed up on my radar, and soon enough I found myself tracking down Cynthia Rowland, a powerhouse facial-fitness trainer. Part sports coach, part motivational speaker, Rowland says she's on a mission to save women from the surgeon's knife (and injections or anything that hurts or costs a lot of money, except her one-on-one coaching sessions, which start at $65 per fifteen-minute segment). As she told a seminar audience: "Plastic surgeons want you to believe you have to use surgery to cut into perfectly healthy tissue to get your face to look young again. They are wrong. My name is Cynthia Rowland and I am on an antiaging mission."

Rowland lives in Southern California, but she happened to be coming to the East Coast and agreed to meet me for a workout session—*if* I vowed to do her resistance-training exercises in preparation. She wanted my face, if not buff, at least in decent condition. As she proselytized about the remarkable improvement possible with her routine, I sincerely believed I'd do the facial aerobics she prescribed. "I'll work out night and day," I vowed. And I intended to, really, except that when her "Facial Magic" DVD arrived, with its rigorous jowl and nasolabial-fold routines, I was so intimidated that I stashed it away and repaired to the bathroom to apply an extra dose of antiwrinkle formula.

"Your face," Ken observed, "is a couch potato."

During our phone conversation, Rowland told me that I'd never be able to guess her age when we met. "And if you do," she said, "I won't admit it." In person, she did indeed prove to be ageless—and in possession of the most (the only?) muscular forehead I'd ever seen. "Feel it," she ordered, flexing her brow.

I didn't confess this to Rowland, but I'd gone into our workout session a skeptic. I know practitioners claim it works, but doctors are always pointing out that facial exercises don't have the power to remove fatty deposits or make skin tighter, as face-lifts do. And medical opinions aside, doesn't the Rogaine principle apply? You know—if it really worked, no one would be bald.

And yet, here was Rowland in front of me, apparently living proof that your face can be a hard body—a gym rat. (I say "apparently" because although I have absolutely no reason to distrust Rowland—zero—in the wake of a shocking *New York* magazine scoop reporting that some personal trainers actually used liposuction to supplement their workouts, you can never be too believing.) She slipped on her trademark immaculate white gloves in preparation for putting my face through its paces. "Have you been doing the exercises?" The truth? I hadn't lifted a lip except to complain to friends about how much work was involved. "Not religiously," I said. Atheistically would be more like it.

Cynthia was not pleased. "Then your face will feel this tomorrow morning," she snapped. She positioned herself behind me in the alarmingly well-lit bathroom that served as our gym, and used her gloved fingers to anchor my various facial muscles as I pushed against her. She explained that because facial muscles attach to bone on only one end, in order to adequately exercise them "we must first create an artificial anchor with our fingertips or even our tongue so that a contraction can impact the muscles so they reposition and lift up and back into the hairline."

I did an antiwattle exercise that involved sticking my chin out, flattening my tongue to the roof of my mouth, tensing my neck, holding the contraction, repeating, and wondering if I'd rather just live with a wattle. With Cynthia's strong fingers and thumbs positioned near my hairline and just above the temples, we also worked my forehead (the lazy bum), and then it was time for the showstopper: her famous instant eye-lift: Rowland put the middle fingers of each of her hands beneath my brows, pushed up and out, and asked me to press my forehead down, against her. I was to hold the contraction for five seconds the first time, and ten for subsequent repetitions.

I was about to beg for a break when I looked in the mirror and noticed—could it be?—that my eyes looked more awake and open wider, as if I'd had a brow-lift. Was my face higher? So it seemed. I was ready to volunteer to star in one of Rowland's infomercials. "If you do these exercises regularly, they'll stay like that," she said. She mentioned that in its unexercised state, my forehead was "mushy." Mushy is not exactly a compliment, but I figured that in a few months, if I did the exercises six times a week, twenty minutes a day, as instructed, my face would be a six-pack.

"Wow," my mom said when I told her about the miraculous results that were seemingly ours for the taking. "Have you been doing the exercises?" To be honest, no. I would. I want to. But who has time? The ugly truth about facial fitness is that it forces you to pit body parts against each other. Time spent reducing my crow's-feet means time away from firming my thighs. And that's not a choice any woman should be forced to make.

Once my face stopped aching from its run-in with Rowland—it felt as if it had ridden a horse—I gathered my strength and continued the quest for a non-surgical, non–La Prairie intervention. There had to be less painful alternatives.

There were. Unfortunately, one of them was the yoga face-lift. I admire yoga-doers, really. They're bendy and lithe, and maybe in another incarnation I'll be one of them. But considering that I can barely do a decent tree pose, achieving simultaneous spiritual ecstasy and a reduction in wrinkles seemed unlikely.

And yet, here was Marie-Véronique Nadeau, the author of *The Yoga Facelift,* on the phone insisting that I would see results if I simply bent over and let my head hang down, yanked my hair so it pulled my forehead taut, and returned to a standing position, still using my hair as a face-lift tool.

One hand holding the phone, the other grabbing a hunk of hair, I ran to the mirror to see for myself. I looked nutty, yes—but also peppier and fresher-faced. I had the upturned eyes I'd been longing for, and my cheeks were tighter. Even my forehead looked less paunchy. Alas, my joy was fleeting. As I yelled "yippee!" and pumped my non-phone hand in the air, I let go of my hair, and with it, my facial scaffolding. Youth, so fleeting, had disappeared once again. (FYI: While wearing your hair in a face-lift ponytail seems like an ideal, hands-free solution, be careful, it might backfire: "traction alopecia," or hair loss from the regular pulling, is a real condition.)

To be fair, there's much more to Nadeau's teachings than just the hair-yank lift, so I shouldn't criticize, but if the move showed me anything, it was how much better I would look with a real, surgical face-lift. This is the wrong take-home message, I know.

But I wasn't the only one judging others' exercise routines. Nadeau, who teaches a yoga face-lift class in the Bay Area in California, had a word to say about *my* bias toward the gym (the regular one, for your body). If I have time for any exercise, she said, it should be lavished on muscles people actually see—in the face and neck—and not on those usually covered by clothing. In fact the gym can *cause* wrinkles, she warned. "The scowls and other horrible expressions" you make while doing crunches "make you look older by the minute." And all this time I'd been trying to stay away from the vending machine, not the Nautilus.

In her book, Nadeau explains that "the face is the gateway to the soul, but the stresses and strains of daily living often prevent us from putting our best face forward. When we were told as kids that if we made funny faces they might stick that way, there was a grain of truth [there]. Facial expressions that express worry, unhappiness and anger have a way of becoming permanent."

Although virtually every single person I've ever met in the beauty industry diagnoses life itself as the cause for many of our beauty problems, it wasn't until relatively recently, in 2004, that scientists (real ones, not the lab-coated ladies at the Clinique counter) identified the first direct link between stress and aging. Health psychologist Elissa Epel, an assistant professor at the University of California, San Francisco, and her colleagues, found evidence that prolonged psychological stress and the perception of stress had a big impact on three biological factors—oxidative stress, lower telomerase activity, and shorter telomere length—all of which are related to cell longevity and disease. In their study, the cells of the high-stress women had characteristics of cells about thirteen years older, on average, than the cells of the low-stress women. If that's not enough to stress you out about your stress, I don't know what is.

But when it comes to your face, it's not just negative emotions that take their toll. Smiling, laughing, raising a brow in mockery are also harmful. After reading Nadeau's description of how we cause our own problems, I realized that enthusiasm had caused a lot of my facial issues and decided to switch to an expression-free mode. Unfortunately, my new antiaging plan began right when Ken returned from a two-day business trip. "Hello," I said flatly. "What's wrong?" he asked. "Nothing," I snapped. Stress creased my brow.

Considering that there's a yoga class owners can take with their dogs—Doga, it's called—I probably don't need to tell you that Nadeau's yoga face-lift class is not the only one of its kind. Similar classes are offered in the Atlanta area, Texas, and, of course, New York. I guess it was only a matter of time before a practice that emphasizes mental and spiritual well-being teamed up with the completely superficial and artificial.

My yoga face-lift class was in Manhattan. I walked into the New York Health & Racquet Club just in time to hustle into a modified shoulder stand and get my *prana*, or life force, flowing up rather than down. "We work magic in here," said instructor Annelise Hagen, the author of yet another yoga face-lift book—*The Yoga Face*. Magic. I was relieved to hear it. Skin care admen have conditioned me to live in a fantasy world ripe with the unrealistic hope of instant tightening, lightening, lifting, and disappearing. I'm now at the point where a product or exercise that made realistic claims would be of no interest. Here's something I've learned about myself: Part of me—the part with access to the credit card, unfortunately—*wants* to be fooled. And I'm not the only one. While 84 percent of women surveyed by the Dove company in 2006 said they are more likely to buy a product that honestly represents itself than one that makes false claims and promises, the more interesting number is 16: that's the percentage of women willing to admit publicly that reality is not important to them. And if 16 percent are willing to say that to pollsters, you've got to figure that the real number who want to be fooled is twice that, at least.

Why do we want products that give us this false sense? Kit Yarrow, a consumer psychologist at Golden

Gate University, told me that people want to feel they have a sense of control (even if it's not real, apparently). "As if they have some sort of power over the force of aging," she said. "We're a striving sort of society. We're very ambitious, and confident that if we work hard we can change things. You can see why we're willing to try products in an attempt to change the force of nature." I was starting to feel better about myself. I'm not gullible; I'm in charge.

Thirty minutes into the yoga face-lift class, when we'd yoga'd every body part except our faces, I could feel my brow furrowing with tension. I'd need a yoga face-lift just to undo the lines I'd caused worrying that I wasn't getting a yoga face-lift. Considering that yoga is all about relaxation, I should have gone with the flow, but no way. "Excuse me," I blurted out from my position in the back, "but is this the *face-lift* class?" "A lot of people ask me that in the beginning," Hagen said calmly (translation: many of my students are tense, uptight people aging themselves unnecessarily in their antiaging quest), "but it's *all* face-lift. Every time your head is lower than your heart, you're reversing the downward flow of energy."

I resumed whatever halfhearted pose I'd been doing, and soon enough the face work started in earnest. We fluttered our lower eyelids to achieve lift; massaged and smoothed our crow's-feet; blew imaginary bubbles to strengthen and lift cheek muscles, and looked up at the ceiling while making guttural sounds, in the hopes of improving our jawlines. "It's nice to know you have control over your face," Hagen said. "It makes you feel powerful." Hagen instructed us to blow kisses toward the mirror (the pressure your fingers put on your lips provides the all-important resistance). I should have been focusing on strengthening my lips' muscles, but I couldn't get past the vertical lines. I'm never going to blow a kiss again, not even if a loved one is standing on the deck of an ocean liner embarking on a long, perilous voyage. I'll have to content myself with waving. I almost slid into a funk, but then I remembered that I never was a big kiss-blower anyway, not even in my taut twenties. And as my mother pointed out later, "No one travels by ocean liner anymore. And you can't get anywhere near someone leaving on a plane these days, so don't worry about it."

After class, I got Hagen alone, and as the two of us sat on our mats, she explained that every time you're inverted, the so-called sea mammal effect kicks in. Your heart rate slows, she said, which means less work for the circulatory system. Hagen listed so many benefits of inversion—for the thyroid, hot flashes, road rage—that I wondered if bats know something we don't. "Shouldn't we spend all of our time upside down?" I asked.

"You could stop in the middle of the day and do a downward-facing dog," she said.

Even though her book is called *The Yoga Face*, Hagen's main concern seems to be not the face but the body. "Nobody focuses on your wrinkles but you," she said. "But what people *do* focus on is how you hold yourself. It's part of the Western mind-set to focus on the microscopic. Alignment is an antidote to old age. If you walk posturally correct, you look ten to twenty years younger."

This made the most sense of anything I'd heard so far. We spend our time worrying about wrinkles that are a fraction of a millimeter, but the vastness that is the rest of the body is on its own. Truly, my antiaging quest was exhausting me. I started the whole thing thinking it was a simple matter of scoring the right cream, but the more I learned, the more I realized how much there is to do.

As much as I enjoyed Hagen and her class, at my age, I was afraid I'd be eighty by the time the effects of facial yoga kicked in, and then what would be the point of all that work? And besides, dermatologists say the results are temporary at best: "Your face is balanced by upward-lifting muscles and downward-pulling muscles," Dr. Mark Rubin, an assistant clinical professor of dermatology at the University of California, San Diego, explained. "A lot of the benefits of Botox are related to weakening the muscle pulling in one direction so the muscle pulling in the other direction is stronger. You can relax a downward-pulling muscle [with yoga], in which case you get some transient benefits, but the problem is they are so transient your body bounces back immediately." Temporary. Hmm. Well, at least I'd have a new yoga wardrobe to show for it.

If my results weren't going to outlast any particular "rejuvenating" activity, I figured I might as well be lying down. In other words, it was time for the antiaging, firming facial massage I'd heard about at the Four Seasons Hotel in Boston. I had never been to a Four Seasons spa before. Starting with the hotel doorman and continuing to the ladies' locker room attendant and of course the masseuse herself, everyone was so solicitous that I began to feel gorgeous before the treatment even started. That's when it hit me: it wasn't my face that needed a massage—it was my ego. If society's reaction to me is the mirror through which I view myself, a fawning public is the only face-lift I need.

I was waiting in the treatment room when Luda made her entrance, quiet but powerful. After a few brief pleasantries she got right to work, cleansing and masking and hydrating and massaging, and then, much too soon, my fifty minutes were up. She excused herself politely and I jumped up to look in the mirror. And? I don't want to claim she performed a miracle, but it was close. My face looked so . . . moist, so vibrant, so expensively cared for. There were a zillion questions I wanted to ask when she returned for the debrief, but alas, my time was almost up. Another client was waiting. I had but a few seconds.

Luda spoke first. "You're a very nice person," she began. Uh-oh. I recognized this as a compliment to soften what was coming. She smiled, almost apologetically. "You need to help yourself."

Help myself? If she knew me, she'd understand that *I'm* the last person to whom my face should be trusted. "Yes, I know," I said, "but how?" Sweat beaded over my healthy glow. "Some pineapple, a little banana, you can make a mask with honey and pull your face up where you want it to be." It sounded sticky.

Luda smiled sweetly and started to head out, but I couldn't let her leave. "Is there anything else?" I asked.

"No hot and no cold," she said, turning to depart.

"No hot and no cold what?" I cried in a panic. "Water? Air? People?"

"On your face," she said.

I was losing her. "Your skin is beautiful," she added. "I wish you the best."

And with that, she was gone, and I was alone in the lovely Four Seasons locker room, wrapped in my fluffy robe, feeling as if I'd let a genie slip through my fingers.

There's got to be another way, I thought glumly. "Have you considered an acupuncture face-lift?" a friend asked. She was in the market herself, but was having trouble finding just the right person. "I seek that perfect melding of spa and specialist," she explained. A few months earlier she'd gone to a "scary but authentic" Chinese herbalist, who had drawers full of moss and lichen and healing tree phlegm, and she left with a bag of mulch she was supposed to make into a tea. This time around, she wanted someone a little more . . . Western. "I want something that says 'ancient mystic skills at work,' but I also want the modern focus on the superficial that one gets at a spa. Talk to me of chi, yes, but also pore size and tone."

"I like that acupuncture is ancient," she added, "even though there are lots of things that are ancient and not so good, like disease. But there's the tranquillity—adjusting your chi, tapping into your energy force—it's all there, just waiting to be unlocked."

True enough, but even so, I wasn't sure I was ready to have an *empty* needle jabbed into my face. The search for youth may be making me crazy, but I'm not *that* far gone. Or am I?

"When people are under too much stress," Dr. John Zhang told me as he swabbed my face with alcohol, "it is easy for them to get old." I wasn't sure if he was talking about me, but considering that I'd called half an hour before my appointment to report I was running late, and then burst into his suburban AcuHealing office complaining about the traffic and apologizing some more, how could he not have been?

Dr. Zhang, a licensed herbalist and acupuncturist (with a Harvard Medical School affiliation, no less), took my face in his hands. "The skin here is loose," he said, touching the bags under my eyes. Crow's-feet were also a problem. "If we can get it tighter, you will look younger," he said. "The needle can make the muscle stronger in your face."

Jab away! I thought.

Okay, so there's no hard evidence that "facial rejuvenation acupuncture" works, but there's no hard evidence it doesn't. Advocates claim it increases blood flow and the production of collagen. While a growing number of studies have confirmed acupuncture's role in relieving pain and nausea, among other symptoms, little research has been done on its cosmetic properties. I've read assertions that an acupuncture facial can take fifteen years off a person's appearance, but, as the *Wall Street Journal* reported, "One frequently cited study concluded that a course of 20 treatments produced a 'marked' effect in 90% of people. But the research consisted simply of one practitioner's case reports and no comparison group, making the findings preliminary at best."

I lay on the table listening to Chinese Muzak (Muzak-upuncture?) as Dr. Zhang stuck small, very slender needles around my eyes and mouth, and in my scalp and hands. Well, I think he did; I didn't feel any insertions at all; and out of fear my eyes were closed. He turned on a heat lamp. "You can just lie here and relax," he said. Just lie there? With nothing to read, no cell, no iPod, no NPR newsfeed? "Relax"? Was he kidding? "I'll be back in half an hour."

Over the phone Dr. Zhang told me it would take at least two sessions to see any results, and in general you need a series of ten, with monthly maintenance appointments, to keep up the improvements. Each session is $60, so that's $600 out of pocket just to get started—and doesn't count the upkeep. Botox was looking ever more reasonable. After thirty inert, media-less minutes, Dr. Zhang returned. "How are you?" Relaxed, actually. He removed the needles. That "loose" skin under my eyes was tighter: I had carry-on bags, not checked luggage.

Back in my car, I sighed. Yes, I looked marginally better, but I knew I wasn't going to shell out the money and set aside the hours to acquire the Zen face—or the yoga face, or the Four Seasons Face. Maybe in another lifetime, I thought, if I come back as a person with endless funds and without the demands of a job and family. I'm sure I'd look slightly better if I did one of the treatments religiously, or better yet, all three. But then again maybe I wouldn't. The stress of blowing all that precious time and cash would no doubt take its toll—on my face.

9.
Face Value

*The key here, I think, is to not think of death
as an end. Think of it more as a very effective
way of cutting down on your expenses.*
—BORIS GRUSHENKO (WOODY ALLEN)
IN *LOVE AND DEATH*

When economists calculate the cost of "the graying of America," they look at health insurance premiums, prescription-medication outlays, workdays lost to chronic illness, hospital fees, and the other expenses that tax our aging society. These are legitimate issues to be sure, but why aren't public policy analysts also calculating the price tag for the *actual* graying of America—and the subsequent blonding and highlighting and Rogaining? As anyone with roots to maintain knows, *middle* aging ain't cheap either.

Why? Because appearance standards have become so youth-centric that biological aging is absolutely no excuse for looking like an older version of yourself. Money that might be spent *living* life—traveling, taking courses, *doing*—must now be put toward erasing any and all signs that you've been, well, alive. And don't think you'll get a pass for helping propagate the species. They've got $30,000 "mommy makeovers" to take care of that now. An ad for the dermal filler Juvederm pretty much sums up society's attitude, which, of course, Juvederm's maker, Allergan, also helped create. "Parentheses have a place," the tagline reads, "but not on your face."

This is what we've come to: The natural has become unnatural, and vice versa. As a friend who got sucked into the injectable filler black hole several years ago said, "When my lines start to reappear I don't think, 'There's my old face again,' I think, 'That's not me.' The artificial has become more real than the real."

Like most women I know, I'm not trying to look better than I did a few short years ago. I'm merely desperate to get back to a place I didn't appreciate while I was there (idiot). It's almost as if we're houses. When you first move in, all you think about is decorating, making the place look gorgeous. You're buying rugs and artwork and putting in his-and-hers sinks in the master bath and talking about an island for the kitchen.

Then, as the years pass, it becomes all about maintenance. The boiler, the foundation, the roof. Boring
and pricey, yet crucial. To borrow from former Clinton
strategist James Carville, It's the upkeep, stupid. With
an emphasis on "up." Eyes, forehead, brows, cheeks,
neck, breasts, arms, thighs, rear, earlobes—society
tells me they all need to be higher. When I think about
the aesthetician hours it's taken to (try to) raise what
I've got a millimeter or two, I want to weep. But I
can't, because that's bound to make something crinkle.
All I know is that there is not one single part of me
that should be glimpsed by anyone in its natural state,
and that areas that previously required no thought—
heels, for example—now demand professional grooming. Not only does every section of my face need its
own vitamin, spray, pill, drink, mask, cream, injec-
tion, laser, wax, and coach to prevent you-know-what,
but the cost makes Manhattan real estate look reasonable. A $20 "after-tweeze" cream for the turf between
my eyes and my brow? On a per-inch basis, that starts
to get pretty pricey.

Cruise a beauty store and you'll see that no facial
zone is too small to demand a product of its very own. If
you're not careful, your upper lip alone could bankrupt
you. Vanquishing the quadruple threat of vertical lines,
mustache hair, collagen loss, and hyperpigmentation

will run you almost $50 (for a third of an ounce of Bliss's Spiff Upper Lip), and that's a veritable bargain compared with the lips themselves, where the talk is of $58 "systems." And once you're spending that kind of money on your mouth's exterior, why cheap out on your tongue? May I suggest a $29 free-radical-fighting breath freshener? The neck, once a forgotten outpost, has been gentrified, to the tune of a $74 "Microlift" from Lancôme, or perhaps you'd prefer Bliss's $48 "Thinny-Thin Chin," which acts like "a liquid bra" for the area from the chin line to the cleavage. I wish the beauty product emporiums sold a potion that lifted my salary.

Where's the fairness? That's what I want to know. I remember when it came to light that women were paying more than men for comparable dry cleaning and hairstyling services, and everyone got all outraged and municipalities passed laws banning gender-related price discrimination? Male-female equality is great, but what about parity among the decades? Women of a Certain Age (the age of which is dropping all the time) are forced to spend more on grooming than their younger counterparts simply to leave home in the morning looking fresh and presentable. Roll out of bed as a recent college grad and you look cute. "Bedhead," they call it. Try that as a grown-up, and open yourself up to rumors about your mental state. "The poor thing has let herself go. That's a sign of depression, you know." The whole situation is backward. At a time in life when you're busier and more financially strapped than ever— caring for kids and elderly parents, saving for college, volunteering, shouldering increased responsibility at work—you have to spend more time and money on yourself just to hit the lowest bar of attractive.

The situation is seen most clearly when thought of in hostage terms. A twenty-year-old who's captured and then released can greet her family and news reporters with pure joy. The fifty-five-year-old? She's going to face some challenges when she's set free. "Even a few days in captivity would completely change my appearance," a friend worried. "I'd be walking toward my family, and my children would say, 'Dad, who's that woman with the mustache, gray hair, glasses, deep lines, and yellow teeth?'" Post-release appearance concerns are one more reason to avoid danger spots when traveling: Survival depends on staying close to her life-support system: colorist, dermatologist, pedicurist, stylist, nutritionist, facialist, ist-ist. "Some people travel with a doctor," she added. "I need to bring along an aesthetician."

Actually, we *are* being held hostage—not in some dark cell in a lawless country, but right here, on our own soil, in the glitzy cosmetics departments of major retailers; in the lovely spas where we fall under the sway of tyrannical aestheticians; at dermatologists' offices where we go to have our faces burned (another instance in which your family won't recognize you upon release). If there's any doubt we're suffering from the Stockholm syndrome, consider this: We've come to identify with our captors so that we actually pay *them* money (and give them holiday gifts, lest they Not Squeeze Us In).

And we're willing to spend big. While the high-ticket procedures such as face-lifts and liposuctions and breast enhancements grab a lot of attention for their cost, it's often maintenance—the drip-drip-drip of routine preservation—that does many of us in. Maintenance sounds so, well, low-maintenance, but it adds up. In "Beauty Regimens Reach for the Gold Standard," the *New York Times'* Skin Deep column reported that some women in the L.A. area spend upward of $3,500 per month on blow-outs, facials, Botox, trainers, skin-tightening sessions, thigh treatments, lash applications, oxygen inhalation treatments—your basics for *une femme d'un certain zip code.* Maintenance has become such a significant factor that it's even attracting attention from scholars. As Boston College sociologist Abigail Brooks points out, the genius of maintenance (from the providers' perspective) is that it's best when started young. "Actresses and entertainers, including Scarlett Johansson, Liv Tyler, and Jessica Simpson, are . . . starting to speak out about their intentions to 'maintain' themselves," she notes. "In a recent interview for *Harper's Bazaar* magazine, Jessica Simpson explains, 'Maybe after having kids, if my boobs dropped down to my belly button, I would get them lifted. Maintenance, you know.'"

By convincing us that "maintenance" is a necessary part of grooming, cosmetic surgeons, dermatologists, and the rest have turned what should be extras into basic personal hygiene. Even the once-simple act of washing your own face—excuse me, cleansing—has gotten pricey. Product is now required. The other night I was cleansing with an Olay "Total Effects" 7-in-1 facial cloth when Ken came in the bathroom. "What's that?" he asked. "It's a vitamin-infused antiaging towelette with a gentle exfoliant and pore-minimizing features." It took all my strength to suppress a "Duh!" "Is it better than soap and water?" he asked.

Soap? That's a word you don't hear much. Do they even sell it anymore? They must, but that's sure not where the money is, according to the NPD Group. The market research firm compiled statistics showing comparative growth for antiaging facial care products and basic care products. The antiaging category grew by 33 percent from 2001 to 2005, to hit $664 million, while basic facial care limped along at 4 percent growth, hitting only $415 million. Who has time to waste on a product that doesn't multitask.

How much more does it cost to be older? Unfortunately, no one's calculated a "wrinkle tax" or compiled a "youth index." The Bureau of Labor Statistics does gather statistics on the amount single women of various ages spend on the general category of "personal care"—a twenty-one-year-old spends $389 a year to a forty-year-old's $564 and a sixty-year-old's $502—but the survey's disappointingly short on specifics. My guess is that the twenty-one-year-old gets to spend her money on whatever strikes her fancy at the moment— hey, bubble bath sounds like fun!—while her older counterparts are forced to use their funds simply to shore up nature's landslide.

I called experts to get a sense of the time and energy a middle-aged woman must spend to get within striking distance of what she had, and then I scoped out the aisles of local pharmacies and beauty stores and came up with my own "market basket" price, or Cosmetic Price Index.

- An old-fashioned bra-fitter on the challenge of fitting the older bosom: "Everyone wants to look perky," Audrey Berson, the store manager at Lady Grace in Brookline, Massachusetts, told me. "They all want their breasts to be higher. I try to explain that as you grow older, gravity takes over and they fall more. At twenty, a woman's perky without a bra. They put on bra after bra after bra and they all look great." And her older customers? "The breast tissue empties at the top, so if you are putting on a certain type of bra, they are going to be gappy at the top, puckery. A lot of time we have to do a dart. We have our own tailor. The older you are, the longer it takes to get the right bra. We can spend half an hour to an hour with an older person if we're having trouble."

- A fifty-year-old publicist explaining the hidden time-suck of tweezing: "You have to act like a detective every morning. You're looking in the mirror—what piece of hair has popped up over-night? You can do this every day, and then one day you spot a really long hair that must have been growing from your chin for a week, and you wonder why no one in your personal or professional life mentioned it."

Now let's compare leaving-the-house-looking-presentable costs for twentysomething "Ashley" and fiftysomething "Susan":

Ashley:

Washes her face with Cetaphil cleansing bar ($3.99), moisturizes with Olay Complete Moisturizer ($6.99), brushes her teeth with a Colgate manual toothbrush ($2.49), shampoos with Pantene Shampoo and Conditioner ($4.99), throws on a Gap T-shirt ($16.50) and jeans ($49.50) and J. Crew flip-flops ($14.50), and sashays out the door. Cost to leave the house $98.96. Time: 20 minutes.

Susan:

Exfoliates her face with Olay Microdermabrasion ($29.99), exfoliates her hair and scalp with Oscar Blandi's Trattamento D'Alternanza Exfoliating Treatment ($26), cleans her face with Definity Cream Cleanser ($10.99), shampoos and conditions her triple-processed hair ($200) with Dove Pro Age shampoo ($4.99), spackles her face with Skin Effects "Instant Deep Wrinkle Eraser" ($19.99), applies Olay Total Effects 7X Visible Anti-Aging Vitamin Complex with UVA/UVB Protection ($17.99); Be fine Eye Brightening Treatment ($21.99) and Sally Hansen Thin Lip

Collagen Boost ($5.99). She brushes her bleached teeth ($200) with her hygienist-recommended Sonicare electric toothbrush ($39.99), and exfoliates her hands with Thermal exfoliating hand therapy ($15.99). She primes her face with Bare Escentuals' bareVitamins Skin Rev-er Upper ($21), applies Laura Mercier Secret Camouflage under her eyes ($28), dabs on Laura Mercier tinted moisturizer ($42), uses Bare Escentuals' Luscious Layers of Light ($42) to illuminate her cheeks, puts on her lip wardrobe—DuWop Reverse Lip Liner ($19), Lorac Lotsa Lip Plumping Lipstick ($18.50). She dons a JWLA Empress V-Neck Tee ($110) and Red Engine Midrise Bootcut Jeans ($154), both from Bloomingdale's new in-store boutique for more mature women, Quotation, and slips her Masai Balance Technology pressure-distributing sandals ($235) onto her pedicured feet ($30, with tip). Cost to leave the house: $1,293.41. Time: 1 hour.

As bad as those numbers sound, they don't even tell the full story. At the very same time our basic maintenance costs are rising, the price of the perks we covet—from handbags to vacations to sheets—has also escalated. Flimsy shoes, cheap bars, tiny apartments, budget accommodations, and myriad other things we didn't notice in our twenties have become unbearable hardships. Or would, if we had the strength to endure them anymore. There's a whole category of activities we can no longer "get away with" without paying the price in time and grooming: jet travel, lack of sleep, two glasses of wine. Ugh. They don't call them "*youth hostels*" for nothing. As with much of life, the change is incremental. You don't go from low-maintenance gal to lay diva overnight. It happens one tiny indulgence at a time.

For example: Recently I celebrated my forty-sixth birthday, and as my present to myself—yes, with age I've embraced the I-deserve-it self-gift—I thought I'd surprise myself with an organic face peel. At $100, it was expensive, but as a onetime treat, hardly a bank-buster. But just as the longest journey starts with a single step, so does a monthly peel habit begin with a single fruit-acid exfoliation. It's like driving over the inground spiked security systems rental-car agencies use in their lots to prevent theft. There's one way, and it's forward. Where it once seemed insane to pay $100 for some vague promise of looking fresher—Who would drop that kind of money?—what you've done is establish a new definition of "reasonable."

And then you're in trouble. As Manisha Thakor, the coauthor of *On My Own Two Feet: A Modern Girl's Guide to Personal Finance*, points out, expensive treatments and creams are even more costly than they seem. "People are paying by credit card, so that a service that starts out pricey gets even worse when you're paying 20 percent interest on it." How to stop yourself? Think of your income as a pie. "For most people, taxes eat up 25 percent of the pie, and if you have any chance of a decent standard of living in retirement you need to save 15 percent, so you have two slices eating up 40 percent. That leaves 60 percent for everything else. The remaining slices are what you *want* and what you *need*, and what we've noticed is that a lot of the antiaging stuff is creeping from the 'want' side to the 'need' side. And it's scary, because the slices are finite." Yikes.

If those splashes of cold water aren't enough to scare you thrifty, Thakor has another way to drive home the opportunity cost of La Mer. "Figure out what your after-tax hourly take-home pay is," she instructs. "If you make $40,000 a year, you take home about $30,000 after taxes, and let's say you work 40 hours a week 50 weeks a year, so that's 2,000 hours, so your take home per hour is $15. The thought is if you go into a department store and try on cosmetics and see a face cream to prevent wrinkles for $150, is this worth putting up with your co-workers for 10 hours? People don't think about it, but that's the trade-off you're making."

Convincing stuff, and yet even Thakor herself is not immune. For a brief period in her life—before she met the man she married, she said—she "groomed up a storm." "What bothered me was that it was never enough. No matter what I did, someone would tell me about something else." Thakor says she finally reined herself in, but she knows she's always in danger of sliding back. "It's like you're in Alcoholics Anonymous and you have to recommit into not falling into that trap again."

But what if, despite your best intentions, you do fall in? That happened to me in New York a while ago. I went to the city purse-less, intending to buy a $10 bag on the street to take to the book party I'd come to attend. The cheapo bag was truly my plan even though the party was being cohosted by Kate Spade. I figured in the dark she wouldn't be able to tell the difference (and she ended up not even going, although I don't know if bag reasons played a part). Anyway, the next thing I knew, I was in a very nice store called Lederer de Paris, handing over my credit card, about to be $700 poorer.

Or was I? One way to have more money, of course, is to work harder, and yet, the longer hours would take time away from your beauty regimen, and in the end that might not be cost-effective. I prefer to use a system of creative accounting that relies not on the Generally Accepted Accounting Principles U.S. corporations are supposed to follow, but rather my own Generally Accepted *Shopping* Principles (known as GASP), a system of rationalization and inspired bookkeeping that permits almost any purchase to make sense.

Take the purse I bought by mistake. After making my purchase, I realized that while I was spending money to stay in a hotel, it was a relatively inexpensive one, and I could just as easily have dropped $150 more on lodging. In my mind (if not my bank account), I subtracted $150 from the price of the bag. I "earned" some money by calculating how much more a cab from the airport would have cost than the train I took. Another $40 right there. Look at that. I'd knocked almost $200 off the price of the bag with very little work. As one of my friend's mothers used to say when loading up on sale items, "You have to spend money to save money."

Here's another way GASP works: The better your face looks, the less money and time you need to spend on hair or clothing, so splurging at the cosmetics counter or a day spa is actually a smart financial move. And the reverse is also true. Expensive accessories and dress allow you to spend less money on your face, which means that getting a new dress—or a Lederer de Paris bag—is also a good investment. But suppose you want both the microdermabrasion *and* the bag? No problem. Do one first, explaining to yourself or your personal banker (spouse) that while it may appear as if you're spending money, you're actually saving it. Then—and here's the beauty part—simply let enough time pass to conveniently forget about the recent indulgence. Then give yourself a new way to earn funds, such as whitening your teeth so you don't need to spend as much on lipstick.

Of course, you'd have to live to be 115 for these monetary machinations to work themselves out, but just think—when they wheel you out of the home, you'll look fantastic.

10.
Did She or Didn't She?

I wish I had a twin, so I could know what I'd
look like without plastic surgery.
—JOAN RIVERS

I'm the kind of person who's interested in the world around me, eager for information about international relations, global warming, the budget deficit, you name it. That's why I watch PBS's *NewsHour with Jim Lehrer.* Just the other night, for example, Margaret Warner, one of the senior correspondents, was giving a fascinating report on, on . . . I'm not sure. The Middle East, maybe. I was too distracted to hear the words she was speaking. "Do you think she's had her eyes done?" I asked Ken. "A lot of people do." "A *lot* of people are talking about whether Margaret Warner has had cosmetic surgery?" he asked. "The PBS crowd isn't what it used to be."

Maybe, or maybe cosmetic enhancement has become such a dominant force in America—changing the way Hollywood directors cast movies, sucking up disposable income and time, separating the nipped from the nipped-nots, requiring an update to *The Complete Idiot's Guide to Etiquette* (never inquire if someone's had work done)—that it deserves discussion among the Weekend Edition lapel pin crowd. Just as the crisis in the subprime mortgage industry affected even renters, and the dollar's worth against foreign currency has an impact on Americans who never leave their own neighborhoods, so has the spread of cosmetic work been felt by those who wouldn't know a Botox shot if it hit them between the eyes.

Spotting cosmetic surgery and Botox has become a second national pastime, baseball for those of us more interested in the celebs in the stands than the players. I was talking with a friend after the Red Sox won the 2007 World Series, and the first thing out of her mouth had nothing to do with the hometown victory. "Did you notice that Barbie doll with the bad cosmetic surgery that Fox kept showing on screen?" she asked. (I had.) There are whole websites devoted to botched outcomes (www.awfulplasticsurgery.com alone gets several million hits a month); entire email relationships based on forwarding pictures of work gone bad; offices at which the only topic of conversation is Work—of the cosmetic, not the business, variety. Cosmetic analysts, the political pundits of the day, hold forth 24/7 on the Web and TV, pointing fingers at those who can no longer show emotion. Never mind who's slept with whom—that's yesterday's titillation. Breast implants and labioplasty are what we whisper about now.

We've come to the point where Hollywood actresses feel the need to state their positions, pro or con, as if they were politicians taking a stand on the Iraq war or abortion. To hear Virginia Madsen talk, you'd think the issues surrounding the injectables are as significant as the controversy over a woman's right to choose. "I believe it is important for women to talk honestly with each other, to ask questions and get the facts so we can make responsible and informed treatment choices," the Oscar-nominated actress said when launching Allergan's "Keep the Wisdom. Lose the Lines" campaign. Talk with each other about "treatment" choices for *facial lines*? Even for a Juvederm and Botox spokeswoman, that's a stretch.

At the other end of the cosmepolitical spectrum, you have actresses rushing to the microphones to proclaim their cosmetic virginity. Like members of Congress, they want the public to know they come down on the correct side of the issue. Kate Beckinsale made it a point to tell the press she's raising her daughter to despise plastic surgery. "My eight-year-old daughter will point to a woman and say, 'Look! That woman's had too much Botox,'" she told *Glamour* magazine. "She spots them because they all look a bit like Lord Voldemort from 'Harry Potter.'"

Given the almost daily cosmetic-enhancement denials and threatened lawsuits emanating from Hollywood, if you didn't know better, you'd think we were talking about banned substances and illegal backroom procedures. Do you happen to recall Shannen Doherty's response when *Star* magazine ran a story on her alleged "extreme makeover"? This is an actress who had her wages garnished when she was on *Beverly Hills 90210* for writing $32,000 worth of bad checks; who was sentenced to anger management counseling after smashing a beer bottle on a car window; and who was sentenced to three years' probation, fined $1,500, and ordered to do community service after a drunk driving arrest. And yet, it was the plastic surgery allegations that so upset her she temporarily halted work on her TV show and made a special "I'm innocent" appearance on *The View.* "I was sobbing uncontrollably," she told Barbara Walters. "If you didn't have it and they're saying that you did, then it's embarrassing, it's humiliating."

How long until an actress outed for dermal filler use claims she was the victim of an overenthusiastic medspa aesthetician? Imagine the tearful press conference in front of the Kodak Theatre in Los Angeles. *"I thought she was giving me vitamin injections,"* the star will weep as she tearfully returns her Oscar to the Academy of Motion Picture Arts and Sciences, her family gathered for support behind her. As matters now stand, stars undergoing work are so eager to conceal their appointments they'll pay tens of thousands of dollars to close down an entire plastic surgery center to ensure there are no witnesses, a top Beverly Hills plastic surgeon told me. "They are supposed to have eternal youth," Dr. Richard Fleming said. "They never get a wrinkle. They never age." Reflecting on the absolute need for secrecy, another high-profile doctor, New York dermatologist Laurie Polis, told the British magazine *Night & Day,* "I have to be like a priest!" The story's author noted that "most stars would rather confess to alcoholism than to having had cosmetic surgery."

That may be true for actual politicians, too; a drinking problem at least has the potential to elicit sympathy. Accusing an opponent of having had work done is a new way to go negative in a campaign. Over the past few years, Governor Arnold Schwarzenegger and Senators John Kerry and Hillary Clinton all faced cosmetic charges, which were followed with intense interest by a public often tuned out to the "larger" issues (as if there are any). In the 2004 election, many voters who had no idea about Kerry's plans for health care, the economy, or the war in Iraq were quite familiar with his alleged Botox use. *New York Times* columnist Maureen Dowd thought whispers about Kerry's Botox use so important she spent 726 words trying to goad him into showing facial emotion. He denies shooting up, but nonetheless Dowd concludes her "Whence the Wince?" column unconvinced. Kerry should count himself lucky a grand jury wasn't convened.

More recently, after over half those responding to an informal Internet poll on the popular Wonkette website said they thought Speaker of the House Nancy Pelosi had a face-lift, and amid speculation in other media outlets, the smooth-faced sixtysomething was essentially forced to issue a denial. "I hear them say on TV that I've had face-lifts," she told the *New York Times.* "I heard one woman say I've had a face-lift, but it looks terrible. . . . Did you ever think that those two things cancel themselves out?" Can the Speaker be unfamiliar with www.awfulplasticsurgery.com et al.? Like many public figures refuting cosmetic charges, the older she gets the tauter she looks, but perhaps Pelosi and the rest are telling the truth. Maybe if you're rich or powerful enough, your face follows not the laws of nature, but celebrity. As the sociologist Abigail Brooks points out, "on soap operas, [cosmetic surgery has rendered] mothers, daughters, and granddaughters . . . increasingly undistinguishable from each other in age."

I was reading the zillionth quote from Ashlee Simpson's spokeswoman denying that her client uses Botox—is there a person alive who cares?—when I realized that stigma-wise, cosmetic surgery is where hair dye was in the mid-fifties. That's when Clairol ran its groundbreaking "Does She or Doesn't She?" ads. The company's challenge was to clean up the product's reputation as something for only "fast" women or bad girls, and turn it into a beauty aid for respectable members of society. Here's a memo the ad's creator wrote to the art director: "Remember especially that everything about these ads has to come through as absolutely real, straight-forward, and honest. Even the tiniest phony note [will] flaw what we're trying to accomplish." Eager to undercut any sexual undertones, the ads usually included a child. Hmm. Let's fast-forward half a century. I wonder if Allergan's decision to hire Virginia Madsen's mother for the campaign, and have mom and daughter appear together at the press conference, was an attempt to gain an equally wholesome image.

It wouldn't be a bad move, considering hair dye's success. If there's any disgrace surrounding it now, it's attached to those who don't use it, says Anne Kreamer, the author of *Going Gray: What I Learned about Beauty, Sex, Work, Motherhood, Authenticity, and Everything Else That Really Matters*. "Because we've moved from a time in the 1950s when only 7 percent of women dyed their hair to today, when a minimum of 65 percent of all women dye their hair, for someone to not dye has become an almost political act—equivalent to burning our bras in the sixties."

She noted that Clairol introduced inexpensive, safe home hair color in the fifties, at the same time women began to enter the workforce in significant numbers. "I think women felt like, 'Hey, I'm no longer a home-maker, I can change my identity.' And hair dye was a very easy, nonpermanent way to do that. Being a professional woman and dyeing one's hair became inextricably linked and today we don't even wonder why. For someone to call that into question by *not* dyeing can be perceived as threatening." In other words: Hey, who does she think she is, not to conform to our standards of beauty?

Cosmetic enhancement is surely on the same path. The questions surrounding many procedures have morphed from "Why?" and "Can I really?" to "Why not?" and "How can I not?" To my horror, I've caught myself wondering why someone with stained teeth doesn't bleach, or a furrowed colleague doesn't Botox. If you look at the language used by the Botox-Industrial Complex, it's all about "treatment" options and "corrective" action, as if lines were a medical problem. These days, dermatologists talk about wearing your face in its natural state as a "decision," thereby implying that the default position is a lift or a laser or a shot. Given how quickly people are answering the siren call of cosmetic enhancement, I'm guessing it won't be long before it elicits no more speculation than highlighting. Websites don't run "gotcha!" photos of celebrities who've gone from brunette to blonde; pols don't drag out old photos of rivals before they added low lights. Yesterday's hair coloring is today's teeth bleaching, is tomorrow's dermal filler, is the brow lift of the day after that.

Sociologists call this process "normalizing." (I call it a pain in the neck.) The more routine something becomes, the less it says about the person who does it. It's true for makeup (wearing lipstick in the early 1900s marked you as an actress or a prostitute; today the woman who *doesn't* is suspect). It's true for financial snooping (driving to a distant town hall and pawing through real estate records to find out what your boss paid for his house indicates you're obsessed; clicking on zillow.com says you have an average curiosity about the financial situation of the guy setting your salary). And it's true for cosmetic work. In the not-too-distant future, getting sun damage zapped by a laser or a nasolabial fold filled won't mean you're excessively vain, just practical.

How did medical procedures become the stuff of shopping malls? Abigail Brooks blames rulings in the 1980s and 1990s by the Federal Trade Commission and the Supreme Court that mandated the deregulation of advertising of medical services. Those, combined with a speeded-up drug approval process passed by Congress, resulted in pharmaceutical companies starting direct TV and print advertising in the late 1990s. "The privatization, commercialization, and for-profit aspects of our current medical system initiated in this era," Brooks writes. Or, as they say in the ads, "Ask your doctor if [fill-in-the-blank] is right for you."

There may come a time when we won't care about who's had a nip or tuck, but for now, we're not only still curious, but eager to pounce. Why is this, I wondered as I spent another newscast staring at Margaret Warner's eyes. Sandra Kent, an editor at the *Boston Herald,* has this theory: "We want to know so that we can adjust our internal age scales. "If Demi's had work done and is forty-five, and one is also forty-five but looks like Demi *without* surgery, then one can wallow in smugness atop the looking-younger chart. But if one is Demi's age and looks like crap, one can crawl into the breakdown lane of self-esteem and say, 'Yeah, but she's had work done,' and not feel quite so bad."

I like her schlump-friendly explanation: The cosmetic steps taken by others, even with their potential to make us look worse by comparison, also provide an out. *I could look that good, too, if I cared enough and had Demi's money.*

Or maybe not. It turns out that even Demi, with her reported breast implants, collagen injections, liposuction, and knee lifts, can't keep up with Demi. "It's been a challenging few years, being the age I am," she told the U.K.'s *Red* magazine. "Almost to the point where I felt like, well, they don't know what to do with me. I am not 20. Not 30. There aren't that many good roles for women over 40. We have to say, 'I'm mad as hell and I'm not going to take it any more.'"

This may not be much comfort to Demi and her peers, but actresses are making progress, albeit in the cartoon world. According to a study called "Animating Grandma," in the July 2007 *Journal of Gerontology*, "Analysis of three animated children's films [*Hoodwinked, The Triplets of Belleville,* and *Howl's Moving*

Castle], each with heroic grandmothers motivating their plotlines, suggests a shift in the representational politics mediating older women to child audiences." In children's stories, the researcher wrote, "wizened old men traditionally give significant advice and support from a position of status . . . but the roles for old women are far less positively rendered. Crones are usually malefactors (often witches), while grandmothers tend to offer passive nurturance." Think a marshmallow wearing a shawl.

But this may be changing: "This filmic debunking of preconceptions about the aged female body—as either (frighteningly) grotesque, or sweet and gentle to the point of inconsequence—suggests burgeoning new relations between children and older women, most commonly their grandmothers," the researcher wrote. Our human actresses may be losing their animation to Botox, but our animated actresses are coming alive. Even those of us humans not competing for acting roles against ingénues need to keep an eye on the competition, if only for self-flagellation purposes. That's the theory put forth by my mother (who, when I lamented the fact that she lacked credentials to make her quote-worthy, reminded me that she has a degree in psychology, "admittedly undergraduate and I didn't buy the books my senior year, but you can say whatever you want about me, you know that"). "When doing a 'Did she or didn't she?' evaluation of another woman," my mother said, "you're trying to find out if she was blessed with good genes or is just rich and dedicated enough to do whatever it takes to stay young-looking. If it's the former, you can be openly envious of her good luck; if the latter, you've got to shut up or it sounds like sour grapes. It's much easier to accept the luck of the genetic draw than your own slack maintenance."

Under this line of thinking, looks are like money. We envy the trust-fund friend in a different way than the friend who got in early on Google, whom we begrudge in still a different manner than the friend who slogged away at the law firm to make partner. We resent the nouveau jeune as we do the nouveau riche. It's as if they don't have a right to their wealth because, well, they earned it themselves (although, as a cushion in Imelda Marcos's collection read, "Nouveau riche is better than no riche at all").

Alexandra Hall, the editor of niche publications for the *Boston Globe,* attributes our laserlike focus on who's doing what to "a mix of jealousy and schadenfreude." The game of spot-the-work is "gross but addictive," she said. When I spoke to Hall, she'd recently watched *Snow White* with her two-year-old son, and she said she saw in the stepmother's "Who is the fairest one of all?" fixation an early example of our current mania. "That's the kind of awful thinking we're obsessed with: who's fairer than us. It's like high school. It's not that people aren't going to do anything [like Botox or plastic surgery] themselves," she added, "it's that they want to know what they're up against."

And we want to "catch each other cheating" says comedian Judy Gold. (If you're unfamiliar with her work, you might enjoy this description from her website: "a mom, a Jew, comedian, actress, writer, author, and oh—my mother's favorite—a lesbian"). "We're all cheaters, and we love catching others cheating," she said. Then she imagined a conversation: "Oh, she's beautiful." "Yeah, but she's not really as beautiful as she looks because she's had work done." Maybe we should make cosmetic dopers wear scarlet asterisks. Or force those who've had work to list their names with a national registry, available for all to see.

This concept that bought beauty doesn't "count" as much as natural beauty was one I heard repeatedly. But why does it matter how someone comes by her looks? Isn't the end result—what we see before us—all that matters? No, according to Laurie Essig, an assistant professor of sociology and anthropology at Middlebury College. She told me the people thought to "deserve" beauty are those who have it naturally, or who work really really hard for it. In the first category are those women who are born lovely by standards set in the Victorian era, when "ladies" had pale skin and child-like or angelic features. Women not thought to warrant beauty are those who use what were once considered "the artificial charms of working-class women," Essig explained. The second group lucky enough to merit good looks are those who put "legitimate" effort into self-improvement. "If you knew someone who struggled with weight and dieted, you'd say she works hard at staying thin," Essig said. "But if you knew someone who had liposuction, it would be 'cheating.' It wouldn't involve that American Protestant ethic of working hard and deserving it."

Similarly, Sander Gilman, the social and cultural historian and author of multiple books on the history of cosmetic surgery, says our sense of who's entitled to beauty has to do with "the notion of the select. This is a very Western or Calvinist notion—that God selects people in very special ways for either punishment or rewards. If you're a bad person, you get sick; if you're a good person, you get wealth. There are whole churches today built on this notion. We have this very interesting problem in the West, which says that beauty and goodness are equal—that if you're beautiful you're healthy, and if you're healthy you're good."

But if you're vain, he adds, the belief is that you're less morally good. And, of course, "only people who are less morally good are going to try and enhance themselves. It's a very circular argument." The belief that "you should keep the face God gives you—that's who you are—says we want a society in which everyone knows his place," Gilman said. That line of reasoning has a long history. "The first time that argument appears with any emphasis," Gilman told me, "was in 1560 or 1570. We've had the first wave of a syphilis epidemic in Europe. One of the first signs is the collapse of the nose, and there are procedures that are introduced to reconstitute the missing nose so that nobody knows you've had syphilis. Well, the church says this is a bad procedure—we know what caused it, and it's a sign of moral corruption, and if you try to disguise that, it's a bad thing."

Fast-forward to the next millennium, when nose jobs are so common as to not warrant discussion, and the question becomes how natural do you have to be to be natural? Where do we draw the line that separates grooming and personal care from cheating? When I mentioned the question to Anita Diamant, the author of *The Red Tent* and coauthor of *A Little Work*, a comedic play about marriage, best friends, and facing fifty, she wondered if coloring her hair meant she was "cheating" on friends who are gray. "Am I betraying them?" And what about me? I thought. I feel pitiful because I haven't done any minimally invasive procedures, and yet I've whitened my teeth. Maybe the lesson is: Let she who is without a home exfoliating kit cast the first stone.

As for those who "deserve" beauty, apparently no one feels that sense of entitlement more strongly than the beautiful themselves. "I have had people come into my office who have always been pretty all their lives," Dr. Tina Alster, Washington, D.C.'s rock-star dermatologist, told me. "They never did anything to enhance their appearance, and now they're finding people who were not considered to be pretty all of a sudden are starting to look better than they do. They don't come out and say, 'It's not fair,' but they'll say, 'I know my friend has had some things done by you.' I can tell they're being accusatory to their friend—and me. These are pretty girls. They've always been pretty. It's their special thing and no one else can do it, and if others start moving in on it, they get kind of nasty about it."

Given the competition—and the vicious whispers—it's easy to understand why celebrities and many civilians keep their renovations to themselves. And yet, in some circles, plastic surgery is a status symbol, a look unto itself. As Shannon Leeman, a London-based cosmetic surgery consultant, told the *Daily Mail:* "[H]aving work done can be another way to show what you're worth. . . . For the sort of woman who lives in an architect-designed house and cares about the labels she wears, getting the right surgeon to perform your procedure is as much of a statement as carrying an Hermès Birkin bag."

Personally I usually keep what little I do quiet—not for competitive reasons; out of insecurity. The few people I told I was using Renova didn't rush out and get a prescription themselves, as they would have had it visibly improved my look. Nothing's more insulting than revealing your beauty secret to an indifferent audience. Meanwhile, after talking to enough experts, and my mother, I finally understood why we all care so much, yet I was no closer to learning whether PBS's Margaret Warner had had her eyes done. I Googled her name together with "plastic surgery" but nothing good came up. Just the transcript of an interview the program ran with David Kessler back in 1997, when he was leaving the top job at the Food and Drug Administration. Maybe that was a sign that there is nothing to gain by learning the truth about someone's cosmetic adventures, and that I must attune my interests to topics with more gravitas.

That, or I need better keywords.

11.

The Middle-aged Debutante

Charm is the quality in others that makes
us more satisfied with ourselves.
—HENRI-FRÉDÉRIC AMIEL

I'm not a quitter. It's just that sometimes you reach a point where the smart thing is to face facts and move on. You don't abandon your dream so much as you leave the back door open and let it wander out with dignity—to pursue other projects, enjoy more time with its family, consult.

I have, as I may have mentioned, spent the past year trying to defy my age. And I can say without boasting that my skin is moister than ever. My lashes look longer, my fine lines finer. I've defined my eyes, lips, and brows, minimized my pores, maximized my accessories, overhauled my wardrobe, and age-proofed my diet. I'm so prevention-focused that the only way I'll get close to a sunny beach is on a postcard. I drink red wine through a straw, and I put in my contact lenses without pulling down my lower lids, lest I cause the very bags that got me in this predicament in the first place. I stretch and take vitamin supplements. I floss.

Nonetheless: I found myself dining next to a flock of twentysomethings at a café recently, them with their giggles and effortlessly glossy hair and un-age-spotted chests and ability to read the small type on menus and disinterest in decaf, and when the waiter came over and started flirting, I was struck by an inconvenient truth: I can't get *that* back. No how, no way. After a year of effort, it's true, I do look better, but the improvement's marginal. Probably my mother and I are the only ones who have noticed.

I know it sounds like I'm complaining, but I'm not. I love the age-related package I've got: happy marriage, happy kids, non-entry-level work, ever-growing circle of friends, the confidence to stay in on New Year's Eve. But there's no denying that in the public's eye, the older a woman gets, the less of a certain kind of currency she possesses, particularly in the United States, where the "ideal age of beauty" is twenty-nine—younger than in the U.K. (thirty); Italy (thirty-four); France (thirty-five); and Japan (thirty-six), according to research done by Dove. In the grand scheme of things, flattering attention from strangers is no big deal. The globe is warming, people—who cares if random guys flirt? They're too young for you anyway. And we should all be so lucky to have cosmetic concerns count as our biggest problem. But who can live in the Big Picture all the time? Or even most of the time? In our superficial world, the truth is that youth is desirable, and once that bottle of milk has expired, if you want to remain attractive to the public at large, spring dewiness must be replaced with something not involving cellular regeneration.

But what? To answer the question that's been driving me for the past decade, I realized I needed to understand why most of us are so eager to look youthful in the first place. Here are the top four hypotheses:

The Moonstruck *theory:* Remember in the movie how Cher's mother (played by Olympia Dukakis) finds out her husband is cheating on her, and she goes around asking everyone she meets, "Why do men chase women?" Finally she gets an answer from the Danny Aiello character: "I don't know. Maybe they fear death."

The whistling-construction-worker theory: Which holds that the less sex a woman wants to *have* (because of decreased estrogen or testosterone or increased stress in her life, or all three), the sexier she wants and needs to *look*.

The cocktail-party theory: The high school cafeteria of the grown-up world, the cocktail party makes clear where you stand in the pecking order. No one wants to mingle with a guest who doesn't *count*. In a society that undervalues older people, you've got to have something to offer or you're going to spend a lot of time alone, feigning interest in your host's book collection or patting the dog.

The "Mirror, mirror on the wall" theory: This one comes from Dr. Nicholas Perricone. "When you're young your life is exciting, and when you look in the mirror you're looking at a young person. When you get older, you have responsibility and [looking in the mirror] is a reminder that things aren't as good as they used to be. Youth is where the happiness really was. Who wants to be reminded every day when you look in the mirror that you're debilitated and your brain doesn't work as well? Aging is not a fun thing."

That sounds grim, but there are remedies. Vast wealth, a royal title, or a great weekend place can overcome fading looks. Sadly, given the amount of money required, buying myself "beautiful" is not a practical plan. Relocating to a less competitive part of the country might work, but who has the energy to pack? "Have you thought of becoming charming?" a colleague asked. Charm. I hadn't considered it. But what an idea! I could drink red wine again! I pored through inspirational quotes:

> "Charm. It's a sort of bloom on a woman. If you have it, you don't need to have anything else; and if you don't have it, it doesn't much matter what else you have."
>
> —SIR JAMES M. BARRIE

> "There's a difference between beauty and charm. A beautiful woman is one I notice. A charming woman is one who notices me."
>
> —JOHN ERSKINE

> "Charm is a glow within a woman that casts a most becoming light on others."
>
> —JOHN MASON BROWN

I was so excited about my new antiaging plan that I couldn't wait to spread the word. "I'm going to become charming," I told the first person with the patience to answer when my number showed up on caller ID. My friend seemed skeptical. "Can that be learned?" She reminded me of the *Seinfeld* episode in which Elaine interviews at a publishing house hoping to fill Jackie O's old position. "Those are going to be some tough shoes to fill," the interviewer, Mr. Landis, tells Elaine. "Everyone loved her. She had such . . . grace."

Elaine (gushing): "Yes! Grace!"

Landis: "Not many people have grace."

Elaine: "Well, you know, grace is a tough one. I like to think I have a little grace . . . not as much as Jackie—"

Landis: "You can't have 'a little grace.' You either have grace, or you . . . don't."

Such pessimism notwithstanding, once I hit on this charming thing, I felt as if a huge burden had been lifted. From now on, I wouldn't have to act as if I'd been born yesterday (or in the late 1970s); I could emphasize my longevity. In fact, as part of my charm, I'd exude the essence of a Past. I'd be the kind of woman who might have hosted Jackson Pollock's first exhibit in her living room, or lived in Paris after the war—"but, darling, that was a lifetime ago." I started fantasizing about my charming new self, an "ageless" woman well known as a sparkling hostess and an A-list guest—and even better known for always having time for those less fortunate. I'll have grad students over for dinner and speak French and curse in Chinese. Diana Vreeland, Kate Hepburn, Coco Chanel, C. Z. Guest, Jackie O, complete with giant sunglasses, making an impassioned whispery plea for architectural preservation—these are my role models (although to look at me now you'd be forgiven for thinking I'd set my sights on Lynette from *Desperate Housewives*).

My friend was dubious: "I'm sorry to say this, but you should have started laying the groundwork years ago. You should have been a muse at nineteen, or posed nude like C.Z. did for Diego Rivera. You should have divorced a count but retained your title." I wish I'd dropped out of the Sorbonne, I thought glumly, or been a spy back when they were glamorous. "It's a shame you didn't befriend Yves when he was an unknown," she added. I thought about the famed New York hostess and fashion plate Nan Kempner. She died at age seventy-four in 2005. In its front-page obituary, the *New York Times* reported that she'd been "a glittering fixture at social events and fashion shows on both sides of the Atlantic for decades." Decades. I didn't want to do the math, but the petty voice inside my head ran the numbers anyway. By the time Nan was my age, she'd been an editor at *Harper's Bazaar* and a design consultant at Tiffany & Co. Heck, by the time she was nineteen, Fernand Léger had already told her she had no talent. My future, once so bright, was collapsing like a soufflé. No French Cubist has ever told me I have no talent. I've never glittered on either side of the Atlantic. On my current trajectory, I'll be an old lady in a Juicy Couture knockoff sweat suit, mall-walking for exercise and gossiping about bingo cheats.

Though my steamer trunk of regret was already full, I added this extra bit of self-flagellation: While I was damaging my skin by sunning in my twenties, I was also unwittingly blowing my Grande Dame chances. I was starting to feel really down when it occurred to me that I don't need charm on a front-page-obit level. Like Elaine, I'll be happy just to have a little. I'll settle for even a slightly more magnetic me. "Why don't you become a debutante?" my friend suggested. I imagined myself wearing long white gloves and an updo, and laughing in that lyrical way the rich do, and curtsying, and receiving my guests, with my proud mother standing next to me, wearing "as handsome a ball dress as possible, and 'all her jewels,'" as Emily Post describes in her 1922 book *Etiquette in Society, in Business, in Politics and at Home.* I tried to reach my mother so we could discuss suitable escorts, but she was out kayaking so I read further. "Let us pretend a worldly old godmother is speaking," Post writes, addressing the debs directly, "and let us suppose that you are a young girl on the evening of your coming-out ball." In my mind I substituted "middle-aged mother of two with chronic lower-back pain, a mortgage, and a memory of the Nixon administration" for "young girl" and kept reading. "You are excited, of course you are! It is your evening, and you are a sort of little princess!" . . . "Don't think that because you have a pretty face, you need neither brains nor manners." Don't worry, I thought. "Don't think that you can be rude to anyone and escape being disliked for it. If you would be thought a person of refinement, don't nudge or pat or finger people." I made a mental note to stop nudging, patting, and fingering. Is it just me, or is it a minefield out there?

Unable to find a listing for "Society" in the phone book, I called the *Herald*'s beloved former society editor. As luck would have it, he had the number for one of the Cotillion's cochairs. But he couldn't just give out the phone number of a person like that, especially to a person like me. He checked first, and the next thing I knew, I was on the line with the woman who held the key to my future. Figuring I had no time to beat around the bush—I might miss the deadline for the planning tea—I got right down to business: "I'd like to be presented to society," I said. "Excuse me?" she said. "I'd like to be presented to society," I repeated. I'm not really sure who "society" is, but I know that's what debs do. She trilled (see above), but it was only to soften her unwelcome message: "I'm sorry, but you probably couldn't be presented," she said. What? Why? "You're probably a little too . . . old." Too old to become part of polite society? "What's the cutoff?" I demanded. I wasn't being polite, I knew, but that was the whole point. My call to her was a cry for help. "It's the whole symbolic thing of a woman entering her adult responsibilities," she explained. "We sort of assume it's when you're going off to college." I was going to try to argue my way into the ball or threaten an age discrimination suit, but neither of those would be very charming. "Okay," I said with a cheer I didn't feel, "it's been lovely talking to you anyway." It was time for Plan B. Private lessons. I was on my best behavior when I called Samantha von Sperling, the founder and director of Polished Social Image Consultants in Manhattan. "Is this a good time for you to talk?" I asked. She allowed that it was. "I'm a big believer that charm will outweigh aesthetic packaging any day," she told me. *Yes!* Poised on the brink of freedom from onerous appearance considerations, I grabbed a celebratory fistful of M&M's. "Let's say you're not very attractive," she continued, "but you're charming and quick with your tongue and magnanimous and gracious and you have a fabulous sense of humor and you make people feel marvelous in your presence. They'll start to overlook things. Your prominent nose might start to become 'interesting' or 'charming.' You might be disheveled and all of a sudden you're 'eccentric.' People will see what they want to see. People will forgive shortcomings for charm." This was the Fountain of Youth I'd been looking for. And who knew the trick was not improving myself but rather blinding others? Von Sperling was spelling out the most promising antiaging plan I'd heard yet, but even her strategy was not a get-young-quick cure. Wit, confidence, graciousness—let's be honest. Those are challenges right up there with erasing crow's-feet. If I had those qualities, I wouldn't be in the position I'm in now, cramming charm before my looks give out completely. "Sounds great," I said, trying to speak clearly through my mouthful of M&M's, "but can you spell it out a bit?" She outlined the five steps to the nonsurgical personality face-lift:

1. "You've got to be confident." That makes sense—but it's not the kind of thing you can overnight yourself from Zappos.com. "Fake it until you make it," von Sperling instructed.

2. "Have a positive attitude." Yeah, right, I thought.

3. "Smile. That makes you approachable." I practiced my fake sincere smile in the mirror. First thought: I did indeed look more welcoming. Second thought: My smile activates my crow's-feet.

4. "Be well groomed." I glanced at my chipped manicure, wrinkled khakis, faded T-shirt, and dingy sneakers. "You're so right," I said.

5. "Be polite. That elevates you above the masses. The majority of people in the world are pretty crass and vulgar." Louts!

Oops. That's the wrong way to think. The trick to charming people, I was coming to understand, was to be charmed *by them*—or at least pretend to be. I thought back to Emily Post's advice: "Instead of depending upon beauty, upon sex-appeal, the young girl who is 'the success of to-day' depends chiefly upon her actual character and disposition. A gift of more value than beauty, is charm, which in a measure is another word for sympathy, or the power to put yourself in the place of others; to be interested in whatever interests them, so as to be pleasing to them, if possible, but not to occupy your thoughts in futilely wondering what they think about you." What? Was she crazy? If I'm going to expend all this effort wooing, there's got to be some payback. Oh, sorry, that was the old me speaking.

What I really meant to say is, isn't it interesting how consistent the charm message has remained? Here's von Sperling speaking more than eighty years after Emily Post. "Teach yourself to always consider the other person," she told me. "Be attentive, be thoughtful. People are very shy. Everyone's sitting on the side of the sandbox waiting to be invited to play. Let them know they're welcome."

She said to offer guests food and drink, make sure the temperature is right, inquire what you can do to make them happier and more comfortable. "Without being a doormat." I made a note of that point. I don't want to aim for gracious and hit grovel instead. "It's the way you carry yourself. You have a commanding presence. You're not slouching, you're well groomed and well dressed. You look like you care about yourself—like you have standards. By presenting that front to the world, you've already bumped yourself up. 'I am not rabble. I am worth care. I expect a level of refinement. I have self-respect.'"

I recalled an unfortunate incident that illuminated how I present myself to the world. I was meeting a friend for dinner, and since she always looks pulled-together, I put on a skirt and nonsneaker footwear and carried a non-knapsack purse. She, in anticipation of meeting *me*, was wearing jeans and a T-shirt. "You look so nice," she said, surprised. "Well, you always do," I said, "so I figured. . . ." Unsaid, but understood by both parties, was why she had dressed down that evening.

Being charming, von Sperling continued, begins the moment you rise. "You should wake up with a positive attitude and say, 'This is going to be a wonderful day!'" "But what if you don't believe it?" I asked. "You have to start somewhere," she said. "You have to force yourself to think this way until it becomes so, because you're worthy of fabulousness." She dictated the routine: "The next step is to carve out time for yourself in the morning. Whatever needs to happen should happen. If that's going to the gym, if that's having a cup of coffee, time to blow-dry your hair. You shouldn't leave the house without mascara. It adds a little extra allure, a little glamour. You should not be afraid of glamour." She was right—I hadn't realized it, but over the years I'd come to fear looking my best, as if obviously trying would seem somehow pathetic.

"Now you are committed to conquering the day. You are armed and ready. Remember when you interface with people during the day you are going to be hospitable and gracious and smile. Give genuine compliments when applicable. 'You've done a smashing job with that project.' 'You organized that so well.' It's a great way to go through life. You get so much more."

Eager to start living a charming life, I awoke the next morning and proclaimed, "This is going to be a wonderful day!" Even though Ken was out of town on business and I was alone, I smiled. Uh-oh, I was alone! With the kids. And I'd overslept by fifteen minutes, and now I had forty minutes to wake them and badger them to dress, eat, and brush while I made breakfast and two lunches and cleaned the house so it didn't look like a tornado had blown through, and, *of course*, showered and groomed so I was presentable at drop-off. "This is going to be a wonderful day!" I repeated. "Time to get up," I called out. They burrowed deeper under their covers. I smiled, but honestly, it was the tight smile of an annoyed flight attendant, not one of a person expecting to have a wonderful day. In the end, we made it to school in time, but I was forced to leave with bare lashes, a lapse I would pay for a few minutes later in the grocery store, when I spotted an acquaintance.

I confess that my impulse was to flee into the produce aisle, but I channeled von Sperling. "Kathy!" I called cheerfully. Kathy looked as disappointed to see me as I was to see her, but she clearly was not studying the art of charm the way I was (although she did appear to be wearing mascara). "How's the school year going for your children?" I asked, focusing the conversation on the other person. "Good," she said, hustling toward dairy. "Your boys always look so cute on the playground," I yelled to her disappearing back.

Evidently I needed a bit more help. Who better to get it from than a certified charmer, Miss America's "Miss Congeniality" 1963, Jeanne Robertson, now a professional speaker. The advice from the former Miss North Carolina was to the point: put a smile on your face, she advised, and don't be a pain in the neck. And if those tactics don't work? "In the South, we say how much we use our accents," she drawled in the most charming manner you can imagine. She gave an example: In her professional travels she often finds herself out with groups of women, and if a problem comes up—at a restaurant, say—they'll send her to deal with it. "Jeanne you talk," they say. "And I know what they're saying—you're so charming and friendly that you'll take them off guard. I make sure to turn up the accent."

I was born and raised in New York City and Connecticut, and often speak so fast people have trouble understanding me, but what the heck, a drawl was worth a try. After we got off the phone I noticed a truck was blocking our driveway and it seemed like the perfect opportunity to try out my new persona. I made myself an iced tea to get in the mood, and then, holding the glass, I went outside looking for the driver. "Do y'all think y'all could scoot a bit?" I asked. "Right away,'" he said. Charmed—or afraid of a deranged woman—I couldn't tell which.

My quest continued. It's embarrassing to buy a book on popularity, but it's worse still to remain dull, so I picked up Dale Carnegie's *How to Win Friends and Influence People* at my local bookstore. I glanced through it on my way to the cash register, and by the time I was ready to pay, I felt I'd absorbed enough lessons to win over the clerk. Carnegie suggests you read each chapter carefully—and twice—and boy, was he right, as I learned when I reached the front of the line and suddenly recalled I'd forgotten to pick up a gift. "I'll just be one second," I told the woman behind me as I darted back to the shelves, the way I do at the supermarket, startling elderly shoppers and children as I whiz frantically by. The person who'd incorporated Carnegie's lessons into her life would

have stepped out of line so as not to hol
even if it meant she would have to wait a
longer herself. It says so right on page 8⌐, ...
from Emerson. "Good manners are made up of petty
sacrifices." But I had not yet grasped that lesson. The
woman behind me smiled that same tight annoyed
smile I'd given my children earlier. Who could blame
her? In the process of buying a book on manners, I'd
been rude.

When I got home, I read the whole book, and in case
you're not familiar with Carnegie's six ways to make
people like you, I'll share them here:

1. Become genuinely interested in other people.

2. Smile.

3. Remember that a person's name is to that person
   the sweetest and most important sound in any
   language.

4. Be a good listener. Encourage others to talk about
   themselves.

5. Talk in terms of the other person's interests.

6. Make the other person feel important—and do it
   sincerely.

All this emphasis on coddling others was making me question whether charm was even worth the trouble, but just in case, I used a three-day period filled with parties, soccer games, and a business-type breakfast to try out what I'd learned. Unfortunately, I don't have double-blind clinical studies showing how the events would have gone if I'd acted like my usual eager-to-entertain, overchatty self, but I do know this: I had a better time at each event than I usually do. Why? Because I learned something about others; I left feeling confident about myself since I hadn't acted like a bore; and *I wasn't thinking about my age.*

Bottom line: My life would be so different if I'd understood two lessons earlier: Make every conversation about the other person—until, finally, you find someone else practicing the art of charm, and then drone on about yourself for as long as possible. And wear mascara.

12.
Don't Call Me Ma'am!

Women deserve to have more than
twelve years between the ages of
twenty-eight and forty.
—JAMES THURBER

It's rude to ask a woman her age. On that we can all agree. But *telling* a woman her age? Fire away—especially if she's middle-aged. I don't know what your experience with the public has been, but ever since I turned forty, I've had strangers stepping forward to tell me I'm no spring chicken.

At my health club, a fellow member struck up what seemed like an innocuous conversation only to move in for the kill after a few minutes of chitchat: "If you keep raising your eyebrows like that when you talk," she warned, "you're going to end up with permanent wrinkles. Soon." And with that, she disappeared into the mists of the shower, leaving me stunned and, I noticed in the mirror, with a dangerously wrinkled brow.

There was the salesman at the upscale boutique who ignored me from the moment I sullied his domain, engaging only to swoop in and advise that a dress I was admiring would be "better on someone younger." It was clingy, bright red, and short—and I wish I'd smiled brightly and plunked down my credit card (and returned it on his day off). Instead I mumbled, "You're right," and shuffled to the dressing room to try on a modest knee-length skirt. When he checked in to see if it "worked"—with the implication that if it didn't, you know whose fault *that* would be—I wanted to call out, "I'm a happy person with a nice family and work I love," but instead I admitted defeat. "It pulled across the hips."

There was the Trader Joe's incident, proving that the unspoken remark can wound just as deeply as a barb. Ken and I had detoured through the store in hopes of scoring a sample and lucked into a wine tasting. We were cheerfully clinking our plastic cups of Pinot— *"Salut!"*—when I noticed the sommelier carding the woman who'd been behind us in line, a contemporary

to my eye, when he'd served me *no questions asked.*
I'm lucky I didn't have any more wine in me or things
might have gotten ugly. "So, Pinot Boy—howdya know
I'm not underage? Huh? How?" My fantasy self was
boozy but empowered.

Come to think of it, I have confronted the age-
insensitive. A few years ago, for the first time in what
seemed like forever, I *was* carded. But instead of taking
my ego boost and getting the heck out of the liquor
store, I pushed things. "May I ask why you asked to
see my ID?" I inquired. Was it my youthful smile, I
wondered, my bright eyes, my . . . "It's your back-
pack," the clerk said, cutting short my fantasy. "Most
people who carry them are younger." Insulting? Yes,
and yet, a tip's a tip. Eager for more antiaging advice,
particularly of the free variety, I hit another liquor
store and asked that clerk how he decides whom to
card. The guy looked me up and down and nodded.
"I'd card you," he said. I knew better than to get my
hopes up. "Why?" I asked. "You fit the profile of
a cop."

Some days I feel as if I'm wearing a 1-800-MAKE-
ME-FEEL-PAST-MY-PRIME bumper sticker on my back.
And I'm not alone. When you hit a certain age (the age
of descent?), it seems you're always being judged—and
found wanting. It's like being a bride, but in reverse.

It's not that any one incident is so bad. Who cares if the dental hygienist remarks that your brows are suffering age-related hair loss (as happened to a friend)? Or if the doctor's lab assistant assumes you're in menopause even though you're only forty-one (as happened to another friend)? Or if a fellow Walgreens shopper refers to your boyfriend as your son (as happened to another friend)? Or if a lady in Bloomingdale's asks if you're your own baby's grandmother (as happened to a friend of a friend)? Big deal, right? Well, no. And yes. The problem is that after a while, the "ma'am" pileup starts to get to you.

To get a sense of the scope of the problem, I sent out an email survey and within minutes my inbox filled. Out of scores of women who replied, only one reported that she'd never been insulted. "Either I'm in such good shape that no one has anything derogatory to say," she wrote, "or, more likely, I'm so far gone no one even bothers to comment."

More common were these scenarios:

"I had a cabdriver a little while back," began S, forty-six, "a bald, late-middle-aged gentleman who started talking of this and that, and commented, 'Things weren't like this in our day.' *OUR* day?? Needless to say, my mood was reflected in his tip."

"I was in a liquor store and the clerk asked to see my ID," L, forty-one, reported. "I took off my sunglasses so I could find my ID in my wallet, but before I even got to it she said, 'Oh, never mind, I don't need to [see] it anymore now that I see your eyes."

"I'd noticed a house for sale in my neighborhood and was wondering what it cost," T, fifty-four, reported, "so I walked into the realtor's and asked for the listing information. I told the broker that we lived down the street, but always had our eyes open for new houses. 'Oh, the kids are grown?' he asked. 'No,' I said, 'still in school.' 'The high school?' he asked. 'No,' I said, 'middle school.' 'Ready to move to the high school?' he asked, pushing his luck (he thought he was being divinely conversational but actually he was insulting me left and right). 'No,' I said firmly, 'she's 9.' OK, so I'm an old mom. But still. . . ."

"Last summer, I was dropping Mel off at camp on the first day," R, thiry-four, explained. "All of the counselors were college-age women. I was talking with them and one said that she had just finished her freshman year at Hampshire. So I said, 'I had friends who went there and I visited. It was a wild place.' To which she replied, her eyes glazing over in a wistful, Norman Rockwellish way:

'Wow . . . I've always wished that I went to college in the 60s!'"

"I have a male patient, a little younger than I, who asked me a year ago how old I was," B, forty-one, wrote. "I told him and he said, 'Yeah, we [the patient and his brother] knew you were at least 40.' Many angry retorts sprang to my lips, minutes too late, thankfully, because I'm sure none of them would have been ethically appropriate."

"Last year, when I drove home to NJ with my girls in tow," S, thirty-nine, began, "I stopped at the local WaWa before getting to the house. I ran into one of my mother's friends there who I hadn't seen in years. When she saw me she was all giddy . . . we gave big hugs and started chatting. I told her I lived in Boston now, she kind of looked confused about that. After a few minutes of small talk . . . when it seemed the conversation was coming to a close, she asked, 'By the way, how's Sandy?' Puzzled, I said, 'I *am* Sandy.' She looked almost stunned . . . and I'm not kidding, she said, slowly pronouncing each word: 'Oh my god you're so old!!!' When I asked her who she thought I was, she said, 'One of your older sisters,' but I wasn't sure which one.' My sisters are 9, 14, and 19 years older than me."

That last incident, although suffered by a civilian, is a variation on the "Celebrity Insta-Aging Syndrome." You know how you see a TV interview or commercial with a star who's been out of the news for a few years, and overnight he or she has morphed into this middle-aged person? Or, worse, a senior citizen? *"That's Sally Field?"* a shocked friend said during an ad for bone-building Boniva. It was bad enough when Lauren Hutton started talking about menopause, but the "Flying Nun" battling osteoporosis? It's too much. It's worth noting that the reverse happens, too. If you catch a rerun of a program you watched as a kid, you'll notice that the actors have gotten younger than they seemed during the program's original run. Gilligan's Island's Thurston and Lovey Howell, for example, once positively ancient, now seem almost— dare I say?—in their prime.

Back in the real world, rereading the email responses, what struck me finally was not the rudeness of most of the comments reported to me, but rather the lack thereof. Most of the "insults" were not intended to be nasty; they were simple statements of fact: You, ma'am, are no longer twenty-one. But in a society in which older equals uglier, merely acknowledging that someone doesn't need to be carded because she's decades past the legal drinking age can only be taken as

an affront. And how could it not? Hollywood, advertisers, the media, they tell us that to age—make that to
let ourselves age—is to fail. As one forty-five-year-old
confessed: "I'm ashamed to tell a younger person my
age. It's as if I've done something wrong and they, by
being young, have done something right. Sometimes
I feel almost hostile. I want to say, 'Don't be so smug.
It's going to happen to you, too.'"

Age shame is a problem Dr. Richard Fried, a specialist in the emerging field of psychodermatology,
sees all the time. "If you want to write a societal prescription on how to raise a generation with body dys-
morphic disorder, you can't do better than the United
States," he began. Finally we excel at something. "It
has always been the case that we saw media images of
people more perfect than life, but there was a recogni-
tion that there was them, and there was us." But now
that life coaches, personal chefs, and $2,000 handbags
have filtered down to the masses, we feel that tremen-
dous beauty also should be ours. "What's happened,"
he continued, "is an increasing blurring of what is real
and what is not, and this increasing sense that if we do
not look like that printed image or Internet image, we
are hideous, unacceptable. The cosmetics industry has
always wanted to exploit that feeling of being flawed,
but now it's also sent to us by the medical profession,

which says, 'Oh, I can fix that. I can make you look like a Barbie doll or movie star.' The average person no longer looks at the media image and says, 'Those people have enchanted lives (and I don't).' The transition now is: I can become them." Indeed, with patients requesting specific body parts—Angelina Jolie's lips and Jennifer Lopez's rear are among the most popular—this is almost literally true.

What gives? Don't we look younger than ever? Yes, but that may be part of the problem. Because of the endless antiaging treatments available, women have come to believe—been *taught* to believe—that looking good *for your age* is no longer satisfactory. One must shine on an absolute scale. We're being coerced to compete against twenty-five-year-olds in a race with no "thirty-five and up" or "masters" age categories. And it's a competition we can't win, no matter how toned or defined or unlined we've fought to become. At best, we achieve the "forever forty" look identified by British style guru Mary Portas and reported in the *Sunday Times* (of London): "[S]kinny, worked-out body, longish, dyed hair, tight designer jeans, whitened teeth—the look that says: 'See how lean I am? See, my style is not remotely dowdy. Aren't you impressed? Guess my age. I bet you think I'm in my early thirties.' It is just about okay, until you are in a roomful of it, and then you realise that the look screams 'fortysomething in denial.'"

But who can blame us? Day after day we're told that the "real" us is not the woman we see in the mirror. She's just some old hag pretender, an intruder who's shown up and kidnapped the real you, the one who's inside, just waiting to be unlocked—by a dermal filler perhaps, or hair dye, or a lunchtime lift. Mirror, mirror, on the wall—who is this crone? In this assumption that the real you is the you who existed decades ago, not your current self, author Anne Kreamer sees a "willful kind of denial over the fact that we are in each moment in our lives exactly who we are. We are our authentic selves, real selves, and it doesn't need to be shaped by someone else." Therapists tell people to "live in the now," but the beauty world tells us to live in the past—in the Then. Kreamer's analysis reminded me of weekend tennis players who, having played well once in their lives, consider that their true skill level, and forever after complain about being "off my game." In appearance terms, I guess you could say that I'm "off my look."

Dr. Fried, the "dermshrink"—that's his email address—says he sees "young people tormented, middle-aged people tormented, I see eighty-year-olds tormented by the imperfections they see." Twenty years ago, he explained, "you looked in the mirror and said, 'I look pretty much like everyone else my age.' There was no expectation you'd look drastically different. There was no avenue to go down other than wrinkle cream, but now the expectation is, 'I should be looking thirty (even if I'm decades older),' and if you don't, you're confused. *What went wrong? Whom do I blame? Who do I run to?* This makes people particularly vulnerable for exploitation."

Talking about exploitation: Is it a coincidence that the Mrs. Fields kiosk is right outside Sephora?

"Today," Dr. Fried continued, "a lot of your identity, your self-worth, is tied into that physicality. In the old days, when as you got older you started to look older, the definition of your worth as a person was not tied up in that." People valued other things, he said: "Were you a good mother or father or church person or temple person?"

Time travel back to an earlier era seems ever more appealing, doesn't it? I've got a pretty good feeling there wasn't room for product in those covered wagons. But since we're stuck in the "here and the-plastic-surgeon-will-see-you-now," what's a person to do? If you ask an older woman whose natural style you admire, or a therapist, they'll tell you the best defense is a contentment not defined by your definition. That's the sole long-term solution, I know, but it's frustratingly similar to the diet advice to "eat less and exercise more." Smart, on target, but disappointingly free of shortcuts, and so unaccomplishable in a weekend. Or so I thought. It turns out that Dr. Michael Brickey, the antiaging guru, has a "proven" antiaging solution that enables "youth seekers" to "think, feel, look, and be more youthful." As he says on his website, "My 40 years as a psychotherapist, hypnotist, and researcher taught me that you are only as old as you think."

Personally I love that line of reasoning—my so-called "ThinkAge" is twenty-eight—but I fear it might be hard to get others to play along.

"Unfortunately," Brickey continued, "you probably have a lot of limiting beliefs about aging that are deeply embedded in your unconscious mind. If you can find a way to tweak those beliefs, you will think/feel/look/be more youthful—and live a lot longer. It's that simple." In my experience, it's not my own limiting beliefs that are the problem, but those embedded in the minds of others; they insist on seeing me as a woman in my forties. But Brickey's prescription was more promising than topical Botox, and I emailed a friend to report the breakthrough. *"You are getting sleepy,"* she responded, *"I mean younger."* Ha, ha, ha, very funny, but that was exactly the kind of negative, aging thinking I wanted to stay away from. Because, as Dr. Brickey says, "your expectations become self-fulfilling prophecies that destroy your health and turn you into an old person. After years of hearing comments and jokes about being over the hill at thirty or fifty or sixty-five, your unconscious mind starts to believe it."

And, apparently, sends the message to your face. But there's good news—in the form of a face cream: Orlane Paris's Hypnotherapy, an antiaging cream for women who are in a difficult emotional period, is now available for purchase in the United States, which means your face can send a message right back: "Chill." Because the product was created by both a dermatologist and a psychologist, I thought perhaps it would be a reimbursable expense. I called my insurer and asked if the $490 (for 1.7 ounces) was covered. "Can I just ask you to hold for a moment while I do some research on that?" the associate asked. After a long time she came back and asked me for some more information. She sounded so nice I thought I might have lucked out. Skimming a 2005 *Neutraceuticals World* article on the cream and filling in what I'd learned on my own, I supplied her with additional facts I thought might be helpful: "It's supposed to 'hypnotize' the skin to disconnect cerebral hemispheres from one another," I said. "And they sell it at Neiman Marcus and on Bloomingdale's website."

She asked me to hold again, but a moment later she was back. "I'm sorry, that's not covered." "Not even under my mental health benefits?" I asked.

Next stop: Neiman Marcus's Orlane counter, where I snagged a free sample. After hearing from the saleswoman about how it worked by disconnecting the nerve endings to my face (is that safe?), I slathered it on and walked around the store waiting for the zen to hit. In the handbag department, lusting after gorgeous bags that were way out of my price range (even using GASP accounting), I caught sight of my face in a mirror and noticed that it looked rather . . . tense.

Dr. Brickey's *Reverse Aging: Hypnotic Journeys to Ageless Lifestyles* CD was my last hope. When it arrived I unrolled my exercise mat and lay down. Music of a style best characterized as "day spa waiting room" came on, and then Dr. Brickey's soothing voice. "Today we are going to focus on optimism and an attitude of gratitude," he intoned. "As you continue to deepen your relaxation I would like you to imagine you are relaxing at an ideal vacation spot. . . . With each wave feel yourself becoming more and more relaxed." From my floor-based position I had a view of the area under the couch, which was in bad need of vacuuming. On the CD, Brickey was going on about water and relaxation, but my mind wandered not to the

Caribbean but to a place of self-doubt: Why, at my age, was my house not as neat as a real grown-up's? Why did I have Playmobil figures, a lone sock, and a book under my furniture? "And while you continue feeling more and more relaxed," Brickey was saying, "I'm going to talk about optimism and an attitude of gratitude. You can listen or not listen, it really doesn't matter because my words are for your unconscious. . . . Ask yourself whom you love, feel their presence very close and their love very strong. Think about your passions and how fortunate you are to pursue them."

Finally, a few "Look on the bright side's" later, the CD ended and I checked my reflection expecting— well, I don't know, but not the same forty-five-year-old me, and yet there I was. I decided I needed to call Dr. Brickey and get some personal help for my feelings of disappointment over the fact that at age forty-five I no longer look twenty. His response was so shocking I almost thought I'd misheard him. "It's okay to look like a forty-five-year-old," he said. "Excuse me?" I replied. "It's okay to look your age," he said. "You're kidding, right?" He insisted he was serious. I had to sit down to take in what he said. It sounded so simple, and yet, up until that moment, every incoming message over the past decade or so had been telling me to deny reality. And here he was preaching acceptance.

A man could be run out of the country for a thought like that. "If you are somebody who keeps learning, and has a passion about life, and good energy level and optimism, people aren't going to care how gray your hair is," he said. "They're going to be attracted to that passion," he said.

Passion? Oh, good idea. Is that injectable?

13.

What Lies Beneath

Old age is no place for sissies.
—BETTE DAVIS

I don't think of myself as a glutton for punishment. But when you find yourself driving forty miles in rush-hour traffic so that a stranger wielding a skin-analysis tool can scan for wrinkles and age spots forming *underneath* your skin, it's time to reevaluate your self-preservation skills.

As if it's not bad enough to happen to notice a fresh crow's-foot staring back at you from your rearview mirror, now you can drive yourself over to a select CVS or department store or spa and actually hunt for trouble. There's a new breed of instruments out there. They measure pores, scope out fine lines in embryonic form, and discover vast plains of hyperpigmentation poised to sprout into age spots that would be at home at a Boca bingo parlor. I'm sorry, but that can't be the formula for a happy afternoon—or a content society. On the off chance that there remains a woman left who actually feels okay about her skin, these sessions are sure to knock some dissatisfaction into her. *See, you were wrong to be content. Now, now, dear, don't cry, it will lead to blotches.*

And yet, there I was on what could have been an agreeable Tuesday, hustling to glimpse my facial future. Why? Was I hoping that my face-in-waiting wouldn't be as bad as I feared? Unlikely, and yet not impossible. I thought back to all the times I'd remounted the scale after a long hiatus, mentally prepared to deal with a five-pound weight gain and pleasantly surprised to find I'd only put on three. I felt giddy! Downright slim. Who knows, maybe all those summers on the Cape wouldn't show up after all.

And besides, I thought, or tried to make myself think, maybe the beauty industry is right in its justification of its new marketing gimmicks. If the salesgirl doesn't know precisely what's wrong with your skin, how can she prescribe the proper targeted products? Under this line of thinking, ignorance isn't bliss, it's laugh lines.

And yet, as I sped to face my destiny, I couldn't help but note that the pain of discovery would be worth it *only* if there was some cure. Considering that not one of the over-the-counter creams I've ever tried in my entire life has lifted my face or frozen wrinkles in what I deem a clinically significant way, what good would a diagnosis do? Why find out you have the disease if there is no cure?

And there were emotional considerations, too: What if I had my skin analyzed, eager to confront my issues so I could move forward with my life (while appearing to move backward), and I couldn't handle the truth? Did I *want* to know that in three years I'll look back with nostalgia at the face I have now? Unlikely. If there's any scenario in which it would be helpful to get a precise count of sunspots lurking below the surface, I can't imagine it. Don't ethicists warn about giving people information about problems for which there's no remedy?

Wondering why I didn't just turn around and head back home, I remembered a call I'd gotten from my mother when I was in college and she was the age I am now. She was with my dad on a business trip in San Francisco, but rather than explore the city while he lectured, she spent her first morning holed up in her room's bathroom scrutinizing her face in the oversized magnifying mirror.

"I was like a moth to a flame," she reported. "I couldn't stop myself." The face doesn't fall far from the tree, I guess. Some twenty years later, the same self-flagellating force that drove my mother to study her nose at eight times its regular size propelled me—a working mother who feels too squeezed for time to make an appointment with an eye doctor or drop off dry cleaning—not just to schedule a "Skinphysical™" at a Sephora in Burlington, Massachusetts, but to actually show up.

The consultation took place in the back of the store, and over the Sephora lady's shoulder I could see shoppers fussing over lipsticks and perfumes, cruelly oblivious to the life-or-death drama unfolding just a few yards away. "I like your shoes," I told the "certified Sephora Skincare Expert" before we got started. Over the years I've found that cozying up to the dental hygienist lessens the duration and ferocity of the flossing lecture, and I thought I'd try the same ploy here. Sycophancy is not without its benefits.

The "expert" explained that her tools would count the number of my fine lines, sunspots and visible pores, determine my levels of elasticity and hydration, and measure my level of UV damage, and then compare my statistics to those of other women of my age and ethnicity. This news—that I'd be taking a pop quiz—was delivered in an upbeat and almost offhand manner, and I was too cowed by the prospect of this unexpected competition to question why strangers' fine lines were relevant to the treatment of mine.

I'd tried to get a friend to come along and get her face evaluated, but everyone begged off. "I'm not that brave," one said. "You've got to be kidding," another responded. My heart was pounding as the expert got to work. She touched a probe to my face to measure my skin's hydration and elasticity, and then instructed me to put my head into a desktop-sized photo kiosk.

On its website, Sephora emphasizes that there "is no pain or discomfort involved with this procedure. Experts at Johns Hopkins reviewed protocols and approved safety standards for Skinphysical™ diagnostic procedures." And that is partially true; the different kinds of light the machine uses to analyze your face are indeed physically painless. It's your feelings that get hurt.

Before I had a chance to pull out my cell phone and say goodbye to loved ones, the Sephora expert collected my results from the printer and steeled herself to deliver the news. *"I'm sorry,"* I imagined her saying, *"we did all we could, but the crow's-feet were worse than we thought."* Based on the numbers the machine spat out, if you didn't know anything about me, you'd assume I was a migrant farmworker or a lifeguard stationed at a pool near the equator. "I picked up 347 pores," she said. I grimaced, but apparently it could have been worse. There was a woman in my age group, the Sephora expert confided (probably in violation of Hipaa regs) who has 1,284 visible pores. One thousand two hundred and eighty-four pores—and they were someone else's!

I barely suppressed a whoop. Yeah! Others are worse off than me! Forget my petty complaints about being compared to peers. I was thrilled. "Where is she?" I cried. "I don't know," the Sephora employee said, lowering her voice almost to a whisper. "But she's somewhere. Maybe Florida. There are a lot of sun-damaged people there." I wouldn't have minded hunting her down, the better to stand close by and bask in the glow of her hideousness. But even if she ever was in Florida, my guess is that she's been relocated and given a new name and face—the vanity version of the Witness Protection Program.

I could have spent all day rejoicing at someone else's high pore count, but it was time to deal with my own issues, specifically my fine lines. Sephora's computer analysis counted sixteen; fifteen around my eyes and one mid-cheek. The Sephora woman thought this one might be a computer error. "I'm going to make it fifteen, total," she said, crossing out the line with her pen. I couldn't tell whether she was pulling a good cop/bad cop routine with the computer or my earlier toadying had paid off. Either way, her generosity was short-lived.

"Your elasticity?" she said, leaning closer and pausing good and long for effect. "It's low."

It was like a crowbar to the knee from a rival skater's hired goon. "Why *meeeee*?" I wailed, brow furrowed, my mouth stretched in horror. Even that was a mistake. According to Sephora, elasticity is "the skin's natural ability to bounce back from facial expression." I glanced in the mirror to make sure my face didn't stay in the shocked position.

The Sephora expert posited that my soggy biscuit of a face could indicate that I spent too much time in front of a computer. "It zaps you of moisture and attacks you with free radicals," she explained. Stress and fluorescent lights—both of which I happened to be under at the moment—were also culprits. Or it could be heredity, she added. I decided to buy genealogy software on my way home; what are family trees for if not to assign blame?

When I asked the Sephora expert how I could regain my lost elasticity, I expected her to jump at the chance to extol the store's miracle cures. Incredibly, she only mentioned a few, and even then her sense of decency prevented her from making big promises. My mood plummeted. Being beyond medical help is one thing, but when Sephora gives up on you, you know you're really in trouble. Earlier that day, as I headed over to Sephora, I promised myself I wouldn't let the results bother me. But I hadn't expected to learn I had a skin problem so extreme no product could even claim to fix it. I *wanted* false hope. That's how low I'd sunk.

But as bad as the cold, hard figures were, the color photos she handed me were worse. In some, my lines, pores, and spots were shown highlighted in bright blue and yellow. In other shots, my skin appeared mottled, even diseased. (The heartbreak of sun damage?) The pictures looked as if they'd been airbrushed by Diane Arbus. If there was any solace, it was that no one else would see them. While Sephora compiles and keeps information on pore count and hydration in order to assemble a nationwide database of bad skin, the photographs do not stay in the system. My instinct told me to grab the evidence and start running until I reached a place where molting and wrinkles were prized. Only I couldn't think where that would be.

Mercifully, the analysis portion of my consultation had come to an end. It was time for the expert to prescribe medicine—I mean products. I'd confessed my pending Renova use, so she limited her suggestions to only a couple hundred dollars' worth of potions. She grabbed a basket and walked me and my shopping list over to the selling area. I scanned the list for cyanide (preferably with SPF 15 for daytime use), but no such luck. That, I would have bought. I did end up purchasing Philosophy's "When Hope Is Not Enough" serum and a tub of glycolic cleansing pads with a mild exfoliant. Usually I love walking around Sephora and reading the promises on the bottles. It's exhilarating. In fact, the clothing makers should take a lesson from the cosmetics folks and start printing the hype right on the jeans and tops: *Lifts and slims your rear! Makes flab vamoose! Instantly gives you the curves you want! Lengthens legs!* But my Skinphysical™ had left me in such a funk that I just took my cute little Sephora shopping bag and left as soon as possible. On the way to the mall's exit I noticed a Mrs. Fields kiosk. I bought myself a large chocolate chip cookie and didn't even pretend I was going to eat only half. The cookie made no antiaging promises, but I figured if it couldn't plump my wrinkles, nothing could. I bit into five hundred calories' worth of skin care and headed for my car.

The Sephora expert had gotten me so worked up about scraping the "cement" off my face—that was her word for my dead skin cells, "cement"—that I literally couldn't wait until I got home to use the exfoliating pads. I was doing 65 miles per hour on Route 128 when the glycolic acid called to me from the floor of the passenger seat. Keeping one hand on the steering wheel, I leaned down, grabbed the box, and tore through the cellophane wrapping like a hungry bear going after campers' supplies. Illegal? Perhaps, but let a cop pull me over for "Driving While Exfoliating." I guarantee there's no way a jury of my peers would convict, especially once my lawyer introduced the results of my Skinphysical™ into evidence.

And besides, a fatal accident could be just what the dermatologist ordered; I'd beat my wrinkles to the grave.

It wasn't until a few days later that I felt strong enough to talk about my ordeal with friends, who were dutifully furious on my behalf. "What does she know?" they demanded of the certified skin expert. "The little snit!" "Jerk." "Was she even pretty?" It was as if the Sephora employee had broken into my home, overpowered me, and forced me to submit to her tests, like some antiaging-obsessed alien. But *I* had sought *her* out. "You know they're only trying to sell you something," everyone said. And of course that's true.

As the *Wall Street Journal* reported in an August 2, 2006, article headlined "New Beauty Devices Diagnose Problems That No One Can See," "Consumer-products companies are trying a new strategy to hawk their beauty wares. In the past, they relied on images of beautiful models to sell the fantasy that women could look that good by using the companies' products. Now, they are exposing and magnifying women's hidden flaws to scare them into buying the products."

And it seems to be working, as a senior vice president of marketing and advertising at CVS Corp. told the *Journal:* "I can tell you that when you have a photo of what's happening underneath your skin, you get committed to preserving it." Skin-analyzing machines developed by L'Oréal SA's Vichy brand have helped drive higher sales in CVS drugstores over the past three years, the *Journal* reported.

But they can go too far. The feelings of hopelessness that prompted me to leave Sephora (relatively) empty-handed also struck customers who used an early version of Procter & Gamble's skin-analysis machine that assigned a dermatological "age" to each user's skin. "[T]he tactic backfired when some women were so dismayed by their skin's purported age that they lost interest in buying any products," the *Journal* reported.

I should have gotten angry, but I knew what I needed, and it wasn't rage. It was a second opinion. In retrospect, a friend would have been the "expert" to contact, with the examination to be conducted in a candlelit restaurant, after a few glasses of wine. Alas, I found myself in a less favorable location: a CVS, where a whole team was waiting for the reporter/fool to arrive. There was a "trained beauty advisor," a publicist in from New York, and the area manager. They were all thrilled to see me! But even as we were exchanging pleasantries, a computer screen loomed menacingly on a nearby table, waiting to air my personal version of *CSI: Face.* Soon enough, the beauty advisor was moving her wand over my skin, and as we all looked on, deep crosshatches, splotchy dark areas, and squiggly bright red lines appeared on the screen. For the life of me, I can't figure out that last one. What's under my cheeks, anyway—lava?

As I watched the screen, one thing became clear: More than I needed any of the hydrating, lifting, or firming products on the shelf next to us, I could use some Prozac from the pharmacy downstairs. But as bad as the horror show was for me, its reluctant star, it threatened to be even worse for the publicist. These skin-analysis machines have been accused of scaring women into buying products, and there's nothing likelier to lead to bad press than an insulted writer. She attempted damage control. "You should have seen when *I* had it done." I looked at her taut skin. "Yeah, right," was on my dry, lined lips, but it turns out she had an on-screen issue, too: an abundance of facial hair. "I couldn't get beyond it," she said. "I felt like I needed shampoo for my face." We all have our own troubles, I guess.

Even though seeing live footage of my subdermal devastation was more painful than the still shots Sephora had shown me, in some ways the CVS analysis was easier to take, since it didn't pit me against other women the way the Sephora system did. It's one thing to know that your skin could have more spring; it's quite another to know that it's not just flabby, it's flabbier than average. The CVS beauty advisor recommended product after product, but I was so overwhelmed by all the descriptions, ingredients, and instructions that the only one I could comprehend was the exfoliation kit, which I was told to use once or twice a week. "How will I know which?" I asked. "Your skin will talk to you," the beauty advisor said. At that point, my skin and I weren't on what you'd call speaking terms; it was the last entity I wanted to hear from. And besides, hadn't it already made its dry, wrinkly, blotchy, flaccid self perfectly clear? If there was going to be any communicating going on, it was going to be *me* telling *it* a thing or two.

Later, to make myself feel better, I called a few dermatologists so I could hear them tell me the results were meaningless, but to my surprise they said some benefit can be derived from the diagnosis, and not just for medical reasons. As a website called "The Beauty Brains" explains: "For the most part, [an analysis] is useful in establishing the baseline condition of your skin before treatment and then showing how much better your skin is after treatment." Fair enough.

With that in mind, after the better part of a year had elapsed, I decided to schedule a follow-up with Sephora to see if the Renova and exfoliating had worked. "Do you really want to know?" a friend asked. "If you're doing all you can and your skin is no better—or it's worse—what will you do then?" She was right, but I couldn't help myself, I called Sephora anyway. Well, well, well. Guess what? The torture has been discontinued.

Feeling inexplicably triumphant, I emailed Sephora for an explanation. "Sephora continually seeks new ways to enhance the client experience with innovative technologies and consultations," the response from the vice president began. "The Skinphysical™ pilot program—launched in 2006—allowed us to look at

21st century options in skincare analysis via a state-of-the art diagnostic. . . . While the pilot stores showed an increase in Skincare business overall the continuation of the program was not financially viable." Translation: We didn't sucker enough people. "We continue to offer our complimentary, personalized skincare consultations and suggest you continue to follow the recommended regimens provide to you by our Skincare Experts."

They couldn't fool me—I knew instantly what really happened. Sephora misread the American Woman. They know we will gladly pay to have someone apply wax to our tender regions and then yank it off, pluck out our eyebrows, squeeze our feet into small but gorgeous shoes, and endure muscle spasms in a bid to tighten our collective buns. Heck, sell us products that don't work as advertised, get our hopes up, trick us into believing the hype—we'll show up.

But when it comes to downright cruelty—to peeking beneath our faces to tell us how bad things are going to get, to thrusting the plain, unvarnished truth about the condition of our skin in our faces—all in the interest of making money off our fear and disappointment, I'm sorry, but even we draw the line.

14.

You've Come a
Long Way, Laddie

Men. We are the new women.
—DYLAN MCDERMOTT'S CHARACTER
ON ABC'S *BIG SHOTS*

Remember the opening scene in *Harry Potter*, when Hagrid is about to deliver the infant Harry to his aunt and uncle Dursley, and strange occurrences are happening around town? Owls are everywhere. A cat is reading a map. People are wearing cloaks and whispering excitedly. It's beginning to feel ominous where I live, too. Outside an exercise studio for women, I noticed a billboard that read PILATES FOR MEN! At a "chicks' night out" party I was introduced to the owner of a lash-extension salon and one of the first things out of her mouth was the growth in her male clientele. "And they're straight," she said. A couple of days after that, a colleague called to chat about a story she was writing—about men-only Weight Watchers meetings.

Afraid of what I would find but eager to get to the bottom of things, I went to the Web, and it was all there before me: a study reporting that in 2006 "male skin care became the single fastest growing category in the global cosmetics and toiletries industry"; a story on the *Men's Fitness* website headlined "Nipped. Tucked. You?"; a poll reporting that 32 percent of men "admit" to using women's grooming products; a reference to "Irritable Male Syndrome," the mood and behavior changes caused by fluctuating hormones. That's right—PMS for men; and, perhaps most alarming, the fact that L'Oréal not only had a L'Oréal Men's website, but it included an animated feature that aged a man's face from eighteen to sixty-eight in a matter of seconds. He morphed from beautiful to haggard before my very eyes. That's the sort of scare tactic previously used only on women.

You see what's happening, don't you? The guys are moving in on our turf. Now I know how the Republicans must have felt when President Bill Clinton seized on welfare reform. Hey, that was our issue! It's not as if men don't already enjoy an advantage appearance-wise. For starters, they have shorter life expectancies, so they have fewer years during which aging is even a problem. Combine that with their longer "dating expectancies," the fact that their gray hair is "distinguished" and their facial lines "rugged," and we're talking some serious inequities.

But wait, it gets worse. According to a study reported in *Optics Letters,* male skin ages more slowly. The article didn't offer an explanation, but this tidbit from the Botox website sheds some light: "For women, whose faces tend to be more animated than men's, and whose skin is typically more delicate, these [glabellar] lines may appear exaggerated and more permanent." So not only do men get to wear more forgiving clothing—the blazer, need I say more—but our animation works against us? Half the time we're being animated for *them.*

The more I read, the worse I was starting to feel, and yet, maybe the trend isn't as bad as it seems. Perhaps now that men are being preyed upon by the antiaging industries, they'll have greater sympathy for what we go through. Maybe Mars and Venus will finally bond—over Botox. If we all know what it feels like to be made insecure about looking older, maybe none of us will have to feel so bad. This could lead to older female newscasters and decent roles for actresses over fifty. (By the way, when Anne Bancroft played the older seductress to the young Dustin Hoffman in *The Graduate* she was a mere six years older than he.)

I was getting all excited about how much we'd all have in common, how they'd always remember to put down the toilet seats and be able to find food in the refrigerator, and buy gifts for their own relatives, when Peter Hyman, the author of *The Reluctant Metrosexual: Dispatches from an Almost Hip Life* and a "natural brunette" (according to his website), warned me that a superficial similarity in interests could give rise to a "false positive" that leads a woman to wrongly mistake a man for her soul mate just because he exfoliates.

"You get this guy who is doing all these things and he seems like he's interested in art and fashion and culture and so he must be sensitive, but you realize it's merely someone who's following this prescription." But when a woman dates a man who looks like the schlump he is, Hyman said, she's getting an "honest picture." Well, yippeeee! Hyman imagined the problems that could arise when a woman who's into fitness and health meets a lipo'd man and mistakenly thinks he's athletic. "He seems like he must have a healthy lifestyle but in fact he's had plastic surgery." Not only is the woman being tricked, Hyman said, but cosmetic enhancement is not great for the guy himself. "I tend to think you are masking some other deeper issue."

Of course! That's the whole point. We *want* to mask deeper issues! Guys really don't get it, do they?

Judy Gold, the comedian, sees an issue for women not raised by Hyman: "Already you have these eighty-five-year-old men with thirty-five-year-old women, now if he looks sixty, he's going to be dating twenty-five-year-olds," she said. "Gold diggers are going to have to get cosmetic surgery in their teens now. They'll be putting off their freshman year in college to have work done."

Or maybe men *won't* have it so good. Guy Garcia, the author of *The Decline of Men: How the American Male Is Tuning Out, Giving Up, and Flipping Off His Future—and Why Everyone Should Be Worried About It,* attributes increased male grooming to women's growing financial, social, and cultural power. "Women have been able to move into areas traditionally dominated by males," he said, "and men have not had the same growth. Men's salaries have stagnated while women's have risen. Women have become more equal partners in the household, or even the head of the household or key wage earners. As men have become less powerful in traditional ways, one of the ways they can exert some power is through their attractiveness.

"When men ruled society," he added, "they didn't have to worry about how they looked. That's not so true anymore. What you've seen in the last thirty years is men have moved from a macho mating strategy to a lot more display strategies. You can see this as part of evolution—or de-evolution. We don't know the answer yet."

Perhaps what's most interesting about the discussion of men and cosmetic enhancement is that we're having it at all considering the long history of male vanity. Have we forgotten that Narcissus was a guy? And as the cultural historian Sander Gilman pointed out, the first procedures—the first nose job, first face-lift, tummy tuck—were done on men. "The rationale is economic—if I look less Jewish, less black, less grotesque, less fill-in-the-blank, if I look more middle class—I can get a better job." And bearing in mind that men *are* allowed to worry about keeping their hair, virility, and athletic prowess, it's strange that male use of antiwrinkle cream is seen as threatening. But it is. Consider this attack on "the continuing crisis of the feminization of men in our society" from Debbie Schlussel, the conservative columnist and pop culture critic: "Today's *USA Today* Baseball Opening Day section gives us yet another example," she wrote in a blog entry. "Last year, we documented L'Oréal for Men's new product line of moisturizers, anti-wrinkle creams, and exfoliators for men. They made their debut in a full-page ad in *USA Today*'s sports section. Well, they're ba-a-a-ack. In today's Opening Day section, there isn't just one page, but THREE of the eight pages of the section."

Why is Schlussel so outraged? As she told me in an email: "I don't think the complete erasing of the line between traditional gender roles is a good thing. I don't want to date or end up with a woman. I want a real man. Some might say that macho image is a stereotype and even when it's true, it should be eliminated, but I disagree. I think it's a part of maleness, a vilified and underrated part. When we're not sure who the men and the women are, we're in trouble. I really don't think a guy who's obsessed with night cream is going to worry about saving me from a burning building." Grooming is one thing, she adds, "But using moisturizer and anti-aging serum—and even resorting to plastic surgery to look younger, which used to be the domain of women—is entirely another. It's the sissification of America."

Attitudes like that might explain why men are even more reluctant than women to go public with any work they do, even though the number of men getting antiaging procedures is growing. In 2006, 1.1 million men had cosmetic procedures, according to the American Society of Plastic Surgeons, up 8 percent from 2000. Dr. Richard Fleming, the Beverly Hills plastic surgeon, told me that men make up half his practice—up from 18 percent fifteen to twenty years ago. But even so, if men see each other in the waiting room, they probably want to pretend they're there keeping their wives company. "The Marlboro Man has not completely died," Dr. Fleming said by way of explanation.

And yet, the *Avon* Man tells a different story: one of acceptance. "Women want their men exfoliating," Billy Kolber, an Avon representative, emailed in response to my questions. Why? Because men sometimes let themselves go once they're in a relationship, he said. In other words, women encourage skin care out of self-defense. Part of the problem, Kolber said, is that men don't really see themselves when they look in the mirror. "They typically don't have the experienced eye that a woman has to identify other problem areas." Well, that's putting a positive spin on the body-image issues that strike young girls—it's good training for when you get older and really have something to be worried about. Imagine the horror of overlooking a fine line because your eye wasn't educated! But of course that's not possible. When it comes to being educated enough to detect my flaws, my vision's got a Ph.D. "I can tell you that to this day, no man has ever asked me what to do about the wrinkled skin around his knees," Kolber said, "but more than one woman has."

I'm not sure where it will all lead. I hope not to male concern about wrinkled knees. That would not be progress. Nor would magazines filled with articles like this: "Ten Foods That Might Be Thinning Your Hair." "Your Best Skin Now!" "Look Hot at Any Age!" "What She (Really) Means When She Says 'I'll Call.'" But we probably don't have to worry. Despite an increasing number of antiaging products targeting men, they still make up less than 10 percent of the cosmetic surgery market. And for the most part, guys just don't get it. When I ran into my neighbor recently and mentioned I was working on a book about the antiaging craze, he observed that fighting wrinkles "makes no sense." The lines are going to come sooner or later, he said. "You're just procrastinating." Later that day, another neighbor mentioned a "problem" her husband was having at work. He's forty-two but looks twenty-eight, the poor dear, and is considering graying his temples so his employees will take him more seriously. "It's really hard for him," she said. It sounded very difficult. It did. But somehow I didn't have it in me to pity him.

Conclusion
Carpe Dermis

Youth had been a habit of hers for so long
that she could not part with it.
—RUDYARD KIPLING

They say that when God closes a door, he opens a window. Okay, so sometimes that window is on the second floor and you have to find your own ladder, but still. So there I was, at the makeup counter, considering eyebrow mousse—as if my brows are the problem. The saleswoman extolled its many virtues, and then, rightly sensing a sucker, suggested I enjoy a "free" make-over. Jumping onto the hot seat before she could ask "Do you exfoliate?" (meaning "I know you don't"), I began pumping her for antiaging makeup tips. I was expecting a hard-core pitch for the miracle foundation *du jour,* but she looked around to make sure the regional manager was out of earshot, and leaned in. "Drink lots of water," she whispered. "Be healthy and happy."

I am screwed, I thought.

As she began the laborious task of concealing my dark circles—no amount of contentment can get rid of those—I pondered her message. I'd already decided to ditch the eyebrow mousse and put the money toward Pellegrino and Prozac when I had an epiphany: Even assuming eternal youth is possible, which at press time it was not, is all the energy worth it? Can a woman who considers mascara a chore possibly keep up with it all?

In a word, no.

To achieve that effortlessly youthful look at a stage in life when *nothing* is effortless, every zone of your person and your personal-effects collection must be attended to on a daily basis—slimmed, plumped, pumped, flattened, plucked, fluffed, highlighted, concealed, lightened, darkened. Groomed. To take your eye off the (exercise) ball—to let your roots go while you tone your core, to skip your nightly Renova application because the teeth-bleaching tray is as much as you can mentally handle, to wolf down a trans-fatty meal when you're running late for your facial appointment, to walk around in a stretched-out bra because your time has been eaten up by a search for jeans—is to ruin the entire effect. It's a phenomenon jugglers understand:

You can't let even one of the ten spinning plates fall off its stick.

As I sat perched on the cosmetics counter stool watching stressed-out women in uncomfortable shoes trying to paint on an inner glow, it became clearer than ever that the answer is not to be found in the cosmetics department or the dermatologist's office. I'd never felt so centered or mature as I did sitting there having my eyes lifted with a light- scattering pencil and judging others, and the moment I left the store I called a friend to boast. "I already have everything I want!" I said, blubbering on about my family and friends and work and—she interrupted me because she was feeling nauseated. "Are you starring in some middle-aged version of *The Wizard of Oz*?" Before I could protest, she issued a prediction: "This won't last. I give you a week."

"No, really," I said, "I'm going to accept my age."

"I didn't know there was a choice."

Her words caught me short. This is the blessing and curse of the modern age. Look at all the things we *can* refuse to do: catch certain diseases (vaccines ahoy); have the hair color we were born with; attain things we can't afford (ah, the credit card); be sad or anxious (calling Dr. Xanax); yield to biological limits (twins at age sixty, anyone?); remain an A cup (hello silicone). We have more control over bits of our lives than any other civilization before. "If I can Lasik away my nearsightedness," the logic goes, "I can stay forever young."

The message surrounds us: Here's a beauty industry analyst explaining the phenomenal sales of antiaging cosmetics in 2006. "Consumers refuse to age," she said. Not "don't want to," or "are trying to fight it off," but "refuse." Head over to the bookstore and it's the same story. There's *Younger Next Year; Count Down Your Age; Stop Aging, Start Living; You: Staying Young,* and *Ending Aging.* You see enough titles along these lines, and after a while you begin to think that when your next birthday rolls around you'll just dodge that cake and candles as if they were a subpoena. If Mother Nature can't serve you with papers, you win.

Except not really. If all the promises and pronouncements were true, women over fifty wouldn't still be complaining about "invisibility." On one hand, we've been duped into believing eternal youth is ours, and on the other, we're being punished for not achieving it. In Dove's Beauty Comes of Age survey, "nearly 60% of women globally believe that if magazines were reflective of a population, a person would likely believe women over 50 do not exist." As if that's not sobering enough, the study also found that we worry more about "looking old" in our old age (33 percent) than about "being lonely" (25 percent). Neither outcome is to be eagerly anticipated, but on the plus side, if you do find yourself alone—or, better yet, invisible—no need to fret about facial lines. You can go out in the sun again!

But we *do* want to be seen—to count! And the only way to do that is to change the standards by which we're judged, both by others, and, most important, ourselves. But how? The women in Dove's study fingered the media for fostering negative images, which means it's only fair that the media be a big part of the solution. Let's require news, gossip, and fashion outlets to run public service spots touting positive stories about aging. And I'm not talking about "looking good at any age." We need to take appearance out of the equation and imbue other attributes with value.

As a columnist for the *Guardian* pointed out in an April 2006 piece: "If Dove really were serious about raising self-esteem rather than selling moisturiser, then it would be focusing on internal beauty such as acts of tolerance, understanding and kindness—qualities that all can achieve and that are worth far more than a pretty face. If parents were urged about their beautiful daughters to 'tell them they're tolerant' rather than telling their less attractive children that they're beautiful, we'd see a much nicer society and one where everyone felt a sense of self worth."

And since we've managed to convince everyone that wrinkles equal unhappiness, let's for once get out the *real* story. As in: "Study finds attitudes about aging contradict reality." According to research done by the University of Michigan Health System and the VA Ann Arbor Healthcare System, "Both young people and older people think that young people are happier than older people—when in fact research has shown the opposite." That's good news to be sure—but now they tell us?

"And while both older and younger adults tend to equate old age with unhappiness for other people," the study continues, "individuals tend to think they'll be happier than most in their old age." (That last misconception reminds me of the 2003 Harris Poll that found 69 percent of Americans believed in hell, but fewer than 1 percent thought they, personally, were headed there. Apparently Sartre was wrong: Hell is not other people; it's *for* other people.) But wait, there's more good news—well, sort of. Older people, according to the study, also "misremember" how happy they were as youths, just as youths "mispredict" how happy (or unhappy) they will be as they age. In other words, don't look back with nostalgia because things were never good.

But who can blame us for thinking they were, particularly in regard to appearance. We've swallowed the adage "You don't know what you've got till it's gone," hook, line, and sinker, thrusting us into an eternal state of "if only." "If only" those wrinkles weren't there, those bags were gone, our eyelids weren't droopy, *then* we'd be happy (i.e., younger-looking). But in reality, and with apologies to Joni Mitchell, the line should be "You don't know what you've got till it's gone, unless it wasn't all that great to begin with." Really—were things ever perfect?

The answer, from a survey of my own, is no. Younger women have issues, too. As one thirtysomething told me: "In my twenties I hated my nose and I focused on that as my big problem. Now I concentrate on the lines forming around my eyes and I can't understand why I was so worried about my nose—it's all one giant continuum of dissatisfaction." No one has it easy. Not the twentysomething I interviewed who's worried about her weight ("You always hear that guys don't want to date someone who's fat"). Not the fiftysomething who envies fortysomethings ("You can still pass for your thirties when you're in your forties, but once you hit fifty it's over"). Not the sixtysomething who can't bring herself to say the *s* sound ("Forty didn't bother me. Neither did fifty. I don't know how I got trapped in the body of a sixty-year-old when I'm eighteen").

But here's a nice surprise: The most upbeat person I spoke with was a seventy-two-year-old woman. I met

Julia, a retired nurse, in Maine at a Quilt-away convention one weekend. (I was staying at the same hotel, but on nonquilting business.) "There's a lot of freedom in getting older," she told me as she and other quilters took a lasagna dinner break on a Saturday night. "I don't feel as controlled. The peer pressure lifts." The others nodded. "I don't want to spend my time doing a lot of that [cosmetic] stuff," she said. "I'd rather spend it learning about the environment or peace." "That's much more important," another quilter agreed. And yet, even Julia feels compelled to do *something*. She gestured to her hair, dyed auburn. "I substitute-teach so I color it," she said. "I wouldn't do it, but it's important to the kids." I asked her how she feels about the endless antiaging articles and tips and products and advertisements. She thinks it's "nonsense." "We all have a time line," she said. "You have to deal with it."

Such wise advice. And yet, so very impossible to take in a culture that rewards a taut neck and dewy skin over almost anything.

So what is the answer? I wondered. How can you remain in the game appearance-wise, stay fresh and attractive and appealing—and yet not find yourself running on the hamster wheel of youth obsession?

I reflected on the wisdom I'd heard from style gurus, star dermatologists, celebrity hairdressers, makeup icons, and fitness gods. And what struck me finally was not any one tip in particular, but the importance of making age recede as an issue. The goal is not to call attention to your years—as in, "Hey, look at me, don't I look young for forty, fifty, sixty?"—but rather to make the subject a nonfactor. Lauren Bacall rocks—not because of the absence of crow's-feet, but because she embodies the great-dame mystique. Ditto for Catherine Deneuve (the word "iconic" applies), and Julie Christie (who just nabbed a SAG award at sixty-six).

The objective is to appear vibrant, spirited, and alive; and not as if you're trying to erase yourself, line by wrinkle by furrow, back to age twenty-five. In fact, despite the attention and cash they grab, crow's-feet, under-eye bags, et al. contribute only partially to the age-related appearance disappointments. If what you want is to be considered vital and energetic, your time is best spent on activities that contribute to you as a whole person. Sure, you want your skin to look its best, but you also need to keep current, fit, flexible (both mentally and physically), interested, interesting, and, of course, up on the most-viewed YouTube videos.

It's almost enough to make a full face-lift look easy, isn't it?

Except not really, and I'm not even talking about the health risks, the expense, or recovery time. Drastic action on one part of your body throws other physical shortcomings into greater relief. Hair, clothes, posture, all look even more aged when compared with your newly smooth face. It's a lesson known to anyone who's painted one room of her house: the fresh coat makes everything else look dingy.

With that in mind, here are ten tips that work, and won't break your budget, eat up your time, or make you wonder about your own priorities:

1 ▪ *Exercise.* I know we've all heard this over and over again. And it's the opposite of the quick fix we all lust after. But without exercise, no amount of Botox or La Mer will really help, and with it, your clothes will fit better, your posture and muscle mass will improve, and you'll gain an advantage over sedentary peers. And don't despair if you're tight on time or motivation. You don't have to become a gym rat; walking can work miracles and can be squeezed into your life. Meeting a friend for a cup of coffee at Starbucks? Get your drinks to go and spend the half hour strolling. Need to pick up a few groceries for dinner? Grab a knapsack and walk the mile or two to the grocery store. You'll be surprised at how much better you feel and how easy it is to sneak in a few miles a day. Even a little bit boosts your spirits, and your bottom line.

2 ▪ *Be smart about your face.* As Harvard Medical School's *HEALTHbeat* newsletter reports, "Vitamins don't generally reduce wrinkles, with the exception of the topical vitamin A-based drugs called *retinoids*." So visit your dermatologist and get yourself a prescription for a product such as Retin-A or Renova. If you're going to spend money on a face cream, it might as well be for one that works, right? And exfoliation is crucial. As *HEALTHbeat* reports: "Aging skin often looks rough and sallow because it doesn't slough off dead surface skin cells as easily as younger skin. Exfoliants help remove these surface cells. Two chemical exfoliants, alpha hydroxy acids and beta hydroxy acids, lower the skin's pH level, which is believed to renew the skin more effectively than many scrubs, masks, soaps, toners, or abrasive cloths." Note the absence of needles and scalpels.

3 ▪ *Put on your face.* Give a woman a makeover and she'll look properly made up for one day. Teach her a makeup strategy, and she'll look good for life. The gurus tell me there are just a few basic steps: Brighten under your eyes with a concealer; use a primer and a light foundation or tinted moisturizer to give your face an overall smooth look; apply mascara for a quick glamour-boost; use blush to make your cheeks "pop"; and make sure your lipstick isn't too dark, since that just emphasizes vertical lip lines (go for a natural shade or lip gloss). It's the difference

between passing a mirror and thinking "nice," and "oof—just keep walking."

4 ▪ *Do something about your hair.* All of it. Get your brows professionally done (at least once, and then follow the line at home if you want), make sure your upper lip or chin aren't sporting strays, and then get yourself to a good salon for a current cut and color and keep them up. Hard as this may be to believe, many people are not focusing on the minutiae of your facial lines, but rather taking in the overall picture you present to the world, and hair plays a big part. Find Product that works for you and use it.

5 ▪ *Don't whine about your age, especially with younger colleagues or friends.* Comments like "I'm so old" drive home the *very* message you're so frantically trying not to convey. A sixty-year-old model I know told me she never allows herself to make a reference that might date her. When talking about entertainers, for example, she doesn't say, "That Frank Sinatra is really something," or "Natalie Wood, what a beauty." And never say, "In my day. . . ."

6 ▪ *Don't leave the house in that.* You don't have to spend a fortune, or even wear the latest trends, but don't walk around looking like a frump, either. That means a bra with ample support, and clothing that fits both your body and your life. And should you be tempted to leave the house in a sweat suit, recall Jerry Seinfeld's advice to George Costanza: "Again with the sweatpants?" he asked. George: "What? I'm comfortable."

Jerry: "You know the message you're sending out to the world with these sweatpants? You're telling the world, 'I give up. I can't compete in normal society. I'm miserable, so I might as well be comfortable.'"

As Bravo's style guru Tim Gunn advises, find a "sweat suit alternative"—something that's comfortable yet stylish. Bottom line: If you'd wear it to clean out the cellar, keep it off the streets.

7 ▪ *Whiten your teeth.* This may be the one beauty boost that's becoming mandatory. At this point, almost every woman I know has whitened her teeth, an enhancement that had somehow eluded me until my dentist gently suggested it, and in the middle of the process, when I contrasted my newly white uppers with the "honey-colored" lowers (to use my dentist's euphemism), I wondered how I'd been walking around before. For only $200 or so, you can instantly brighten your look and the results last for years. Make sure to do it under a dentist's supervision so

you don't end up causing any new dental problems that will require yet another fix.

8 ▪ *Don't try to sound younger than you are by adopting teen vernacular.* There's something alarming about a fiftysomething woman announcing that she'll be "chillin' like a villain in her crib, fo' shizzle." And if you, like, find yourself using "like" too much, wean yourself. It's, like, aging.

9 ▪ *Go to sleep.* Like exercise, sleep is one of those free antiaging miracle tools that doesn't get enough attention. The better rested you are, the fresher and more awake your face looks, the less you eat, and the more you feel like taking a walk. Just make sure not to sleep facedown so your pillow doesn't wrinkle your face.

10 ▪ *Work on your charm.* A sparkling personality can make up for a deficit in the looks department. Be interested in others, smile, listen, be engaged in the world. *You* won't be thinking about your appearance and neither will others.

And if all this sounds like too much to absorb, just remember the two basics to a beautiful life: inner happiness and sunblock.

Acknowledgments

When people hear I spent over a year investigating the antiaging industry, the first thing they ask (actually, the *only* thing they ask—not even my own mother talks to me about anything else) is: "What works?" Everyone wants a quick fix, so after uttering the obligatory "You look great, but if you want to do something," I give practical advice: exercise, sleep, bleach your teeth, get a good haircut, use prescription-strength retin-A, wear concealer and tinted moisturizer, buy flattering clothes, stand up straight. But no one asks the real question: How can I make age recede as an issue and enjoy my life?

One way is to delight in what you do, and in that, I've been fortunate. Except for the afternoons I subjected myself to analyses of the wrinkles forming *under* my skin, and the time a facial personal trainer pronounced my forehead "mushy," I loved this project. And not only because I learned where to sit in a restaurant to take advantage of the most flattering light. It's because I had the pleasure of working with the smart, dedicated, and delightful Brettne Bloom, Marjorie Braman, and Dee Dee DeBartlo. Thank you! And Peggy Hageman, Joseph Papa, and the rest of the team at William Morrow, you've gone above and beyond the call of publishing. Deborah Kerner, Kimberly Glyder, and Oren Brimer, you rock.

To my friends, who never ask me for help with their day jobs but who help me so much with mine: Marie Morris, your talent thrills me. Sande Kent, you're a glass of champagne. Jenny Clancy, thank you for being my first reader and for always being so very, very nice. So many were so generous with their wit and wisdom: Julie Boris, Virginia Buckingham, Erica Caplan, Lauren Beckham Falcone, Carey Goldberg, Susan McConathy, Jill Radsken, Jan Saragoni, Susan Senator, Linda Teitell, Mark Teitell, Emily Miles Terry, Elissa Weitzman, Sandy White, and Laura Zigman. Thanks to all for not flagging my emails as spam.

I'm also grateful, for support of every type possible, to my mother, one of the two youngest people I know, and to my father, the other. And to my in-laws, who not only came to every local reading I did for my first book, but who laughed each time. And finally to my husband, Ken, for his editing, joke-sharpening, and tech savvy, but most of all for pretending not to see where I need Botox.

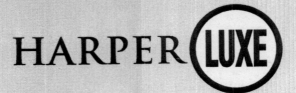
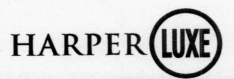